TO SCHIZOPHRENIA AND BACK

By Annie Moon

'One million people commit suicide every year'
The World Health Organization

Annie Moon

All rights reserved, no part of this publication may be reproduced by any means, electronic, mechanical photocopying, documentary, film or in any other format without prior written permission of the publisher.

> Published by
> Chipmunkapublishing
> PO Box 6872
> Brentwood
> Essex CM13 1ZT
> United Kingdom

http://www.chipmunkapublishing.com

Copyright © Annie Moon 2007

Proof-read by Mary Dow

TO SCHIZOPHRENIA AND BACK

DEDICATIONS

Thank you to:-

My husband for your support over the years

To my friends especially Brenda who never judged me as a loony and who never saw my as anything but an equal

To my children who are my life

To DR. D who helped me to get my self worth back

To the people on WWW.Schizophrenia.com who supported me at times of need and encouraged me.

To my good friend Stephen, as well as the doctors and nurses at the local hospital

Annie Moon

TO SCHIZOPHRENIA AND BACK

CHAPTER ONE

INTRODUCTION

Why am I writing this book?

I am writing this book for all those men and women who have been struck down in the prime of their life with the devastating illness SCHIZOPHRENIA.

Schizophrenia has no social boundaries and affects one in every hundred of us.

I am a trained nurse and soon to be social worker. I am also a mother, wife, friend and patient/service user. My book covers all the aspects of my battle with schizophrenia from all points of view including others' perceptions. I kept diaries of psychotic episodes. I have been detained many times under the mental health act. I was told at one point that I would never return to work... I will be in my final year at university from September, doing a social work degree. My aim with this book is to enlighten people and offer hope to those affected.

The book is necessary as there are not many sufferers who come through the other side. The book includes not only my diaries but also contributions from others involved in the life of someone who has schizophrenia. Its purpose is to give hope and validation to feelings that everybody concerned has. One thought that my husband shared with me was that he'd wished that I'd died on the moors when I had gone up there one winter's night to join the spirit world. People have these thoughts and I want to say that it is ok to talk about them.

I want to show people that people with mental health problems can adapt and live with them. I want to offer my coping mechanisms to others and dispel the myth that schizophrenics shuffle around psychiatric wards in between bouts of violence.

I want to promote the positive things that professionals have helped me with and discuss the not so helpful things, therefore promoting good practice via my own feedback on my own personal care.

I want to give an insight into what it is like to have to take the medication and into how the side effects can cause more problems including tremors, weight gain, anxiety, lethargy and the feeling of just existing.

The book will hopefully help marriages and the well being of the children involved (I have now been married for twenty one years).

Hope will be promoted: maybe you won't fully

TO SCHIZOPHRENIA AND BACK

recover but the book will show that you can fulfil your ambitions, such as following a career as I have done with the social work, with the help of the professionals (as most are there to help and not just to lock you up).

Helpful telephone numbers and addresses will be in the appendices chapter.

The chapters will be as follows:-

1) Introduction, what the book is about, why it has been written in the style that is has.

2) Childhood, including abuse and neglect, a relevant road traffic accident, a trip on my own backpacking around Europe aged 17 years being the main start of my psychosis (undiagnosed until age 27).

3) Nursing career highs and lows relevant to mental health problems.

4) Family life, the effect of the illness on my husband, children, parents and friends with contributions from them.

5) Breakdown, hospital, mental health act, police, neighbours, family doctor (General Practitioner), denial of problem, diaries.

6) Recovery including the different types of medication tried and their side effects. The learning curve through denial. The schizophrenia chat room on the internet.

7) Rehabilitation that helped, Community Psychiatric Nurses and their care plan. Support worker. Financial help and advice. Friends.

8) Cognitive behavioural therapy, discussion of how it helped to minimise risks and reduce relapse rates. With a contribution from a Consultant Psychologist.

9) New career feelings about self worth, confidence, applying to university. Story behind cancelling my place, then an error by the university (fate) meant my place was still on offer. Struggles with prejudice and stereotypical ideas including my own self-prejudice. Help from equalities and diversity.

10) Conclusion: - helpful pointers for those concerned including medication, diet, exercise,

TO SCHIZOPHRENIA AND BACK

weight, mental stimulation, baby steps, family, saying sorry to your children.

11) Mental Health Social Exclusion and Employment

Why am I writing in this style?

As a sufferer of schizophrenia myself, I know how difficult it is to concentrate, let alone read a book.
I find written words with headings and graphics much easier to take in. One of my traits is to repeat things; I find that this style aids memory and this has been one of my coping mechanisms for studying at University, i.e. copious amounts of repetitive notes with bullet points etc.

Who is this book for?

- ✓ SUFFERERS
- ✓ FAMILY
- ✓ FRIENDS
- ✓ SOCIAL WORKERS
- ✓ PSYCHOLOGISTS
- ✓ COUNSELLORS

Annie Moon

- ✓ GENERAL PRACTITIONERS
- ✓ COMMUNITY PSYCHIATRIC NURSES
- ✓ MENTAL HEALTH WORKERS
- ✓ OCCUPATIONAL THERAPISTS
- ✓ PSYCHIATRISTS

<u>What is my message?</u>

I want to let all those people, whose lives have been turned upside down, know that, no matter how bad things get, there is always light at the end of the tunnel!

I hope that my story will help other sufferers to come to terms with their situation and I hope that you will all use your own special individual talents, skills and abilities in every day life. Your qualities tend to be forgotten about or pushed to one side when you are given the diagnosis of schizophrenia.

Later in the book I will include some extracts from the diaries that I kept during my psychoses. These diaries were my way of coping and were also of benefit to the health care workers in understanding what was going on in my mind.

First I would like to tell you a bit about myself. In chapter two I discuss my upbringing throughout childhood and some of my adventures in Europe.

TO SCHIZOPHRENIA AND BACK

CHAPTER TWO

BACKGROUND

I was born in a terraced house on a cobbled stone street in 1967. Nobody on the street had a car except for our family, so we were considered quite posh. Dad had his own business as a haulage contractor and mum was a singer with many strings to her bow; she could bake, cut hair and sew as well as being an excellent rock'n'roll dancer. 13 months after I was born my youngest brother came along. Mum said that when he was delivered the midwife began screaming and the next thing my mum knew the midwife had committed suicide after falling out with her lesbian lover. (Well that's mum's version anyway!)

Altogether there was my eldest brother Nobby, 7 years my senior, then my sister 5 years older than me, myself and my younger brother by 13 months.

I will not go into any sordid details about the whys and wherefores of Mum and Dad's marriage break-up; needless to say it was acrimonious on Mum's part.

Mum saved up secretly and bought a run down house, which Dad did up in terms of renovation, and he built a bathroom extension. The house was absolutely lovely when it was completed and

Annie Moon

was one big adventure for us children - I was 8 at the time.

Mum said that Dad would join us when he had sold the terraced house. The months went by; Dad never did join us; it was all one big lie. I later found out that Nobby, my eldest brother, was left at school only to arrive home at the terraced house to find that his mother and siblings had left not only the house, but himself also.

Dad's house was eventually subject to a compulsory purchase order and was condemned as unsafe and the houses on the whole street were demolished; now there are what I call 'Lego' houses where ours once stood.

At the new house the first couple of years were great and there were lots of people coming and going. Mum had some nice boyfriends although life was eventful at our house; life was not 'normal'.

One of Mum's boyfriends was a lovely man who helped me to pass my 11+. She kept moving him in and then throwing him out. There would be a busted suitcase regularly spilling out clothes in the front garden. Although I liked this man he assaulted my Dad with part of a paving stone and I remember Dad having an enormous 'shiner' of a black eye.

This particular boyfriend had a son who moved in

TO SCHIZOPHRENIA AND BACK

briefly. My sister had a friend who needed a home so Mum temporarily fostered her, so our house was 'lively' to say the least: just imagine it - teenage girls and boys together, not related and related. I feel that these details should be left to the imagination as this book is not meant to cause distress to anyone, quite the opposite.

My older sister would often baby sit for my brother and I; looking back now, I was eight and she was only thirteen at the time. Mum would be out singing in the night clubs, my sister would have us in bed at 7pm and would go hysterical if we came down stairs, and needless to say I was petrified of her. I needed the toilet downstairs one evening but was so afraid that I opened my bowels in some newspaper and put it in the toy box. It was quite a while before anyone discovered what the smell was!

Mum stamped on my sister's head on the kitchen floor, my sister went to live at Dads, my sister was probably still only thirteen at the time, it was horrible. Mum would try to poison our minds against my sister and Dad by being manipulative, saying that my sister would only see me to show off her new clothes that 'daddy' had bought her. My Mum was a real nasty piece of work, yet to the outside world she was funny and charming and friends would often say 'ooh I wish she was my mum' - I never ever discussed the violence, aggression, mental cruelty and drinking to anybody, mainly because I thought it was normal and not very interesting to talk about.

My younger brother was a rogue to say the least and was put into council care when he was about ten. I was so jealous that I wanted to be in care, he seemed to be really enjoying it from the stories about the activities that he took part in and the attention that he got from his social worker.

The house was emptied of people one by one leaving Mum and me alone. She began drinking and became alcoholic. There was one occasion when I lost my contact lens after I had had it in my mouth. I would have been about twelve years old. Mum gave me a sieve and a spoon and made me sieve my faeces. She would have terrible mood swings, she would stay in bed all day or lie on the couch, she was violent towards my siblings. At one time I thought she was going to stab me. Alcoholism is a terribly destructive disease and as a child you have nothing to compare such behaviour to as you think that it is 'normal'. I was scared of Mum. I am not scared of her now as she is an old lady, 'pitiful' really. (She has since been diagnosed as having Bipolar disorder, also known as manic depression).

My younger brother had an upset stomach and diarrhoea on one occasion and Mum was in the bathroom. He opened the toilet door, which hadn't been locked. Mum became very angry; he wasn't

TO SCHIZOPHRENIA AND BACK

allowed on the toilet at that moment and had diarrhoea on the passageway floor. Mum battered him for that and the fact that he opened the door whilst she was in the bathroom.

Mum was left. There were other boyfriends, all very nice people, but not my dad.

SCHOOL DAYS

My first 'spiritual' feeling was the first day at infants' school. I was 5 years old at the time. There was thick fog and extremely poor visibility, probably up to no more than 2 metres around me. I was on the school playing field. I felt totally isolated except for the distant voices of the other children in the playground.

School for me was very pleasurable. During my early years I strived to compete academically with my peers. I was, however, very average when it came to intelligence.

When we moved away from the terraced house, I had to start a new school. I was 8 years old and the children at the new school had already bonded into their social groups. At a new school, with a different accent from the other children, I made friends but it was not the same. Everybody was more concerned with why my younger brother wasn't at school and the headmaster often took me with him, back to our house, to get my brother who would be home alone at 7 years old.

My Mum's boyfriend helped me to pass my exams to get into grammar school. My Dad bought me a huge cuddly dog which I called Brian. I loved that stuffed toy.

Grammar school started off as a nightmare; with everything going on at home and none of my primary school friends at the same school as me, not to mention that I was not emotionally mature enough for 'big' school, I changed.

I began having deja vu experiences at 11 years old. They happened when I was in the bathroom; I would feel as if I was reliving my actions and thoughts from a previous time. It also happened at school.

The school was very old and I remember walking down a corridor and feeling physically nauseous and faint due to what I thought were premonitions. I was also overcome with a feeling of coldness.

At about this age I had my lovely long hair cut to the then fashionable 'feather cut' and I discovered that I needed glasses. My 'nickname' was 'Joe 90'. This really upset me because I had never watched the program on television and I didn't take it in good humour. Years later I'd joke about it with my husband, who often calls me 'Joe 90' when I have got my glasses on. My modern

TO SCHIZOPHRENIA AND BACK

glasses are not nearly as thick and large as the ones I had back then!

Throughout the rest of my compulsory school years I was a troubled soul, not only emotionally because of my home life, but also academically- I rarely did homework because I was always getting the work out but never getting anywhere with it. If I couldn't do it I wouldn't ask for help; how could I with mum always 'ill'? The good intention on my part to do the homework was there, but I just couldn't get organised. I was always overwhelmed with the tasks at hand.

I did have a couple of devastatingly emotional upsets, both over pet dogs. These events are part of the reason that I won't have anything other than goldfish for pets (even they are a worry, what with feeding them, cleaning them and treating their ailments!)

The first upset was with a mongrel puppy that my Mum bought. It started to get sick with distemper; it was such an upsetting sight to see. The poor puppy was so ill and in need of veterinary attention. Mum told me to speak to my Dad as she was on the couch and would not take it to the vets. Eventually I took the dog, wrapped up in a blanket, on two busses to the vets; I would have been 12 years old. The vet gave me some medication for him and said that he was unlikely to

Annie Moon

recover.

The following week whilst I was at school, Mum took the dog back to the vets and had him put to sleep.

The second heartbreaker was when a rough collie that I had named 'Lady' was run over. I trained her to do tricks, she was a beautiful dog. Mum let her out to wander the streets (our new home was on a main road, which was very busy). Luckily at the time Mum had a lovely, wealthy boyfriend who paid for Lady's veterinary care. Lady had a fractured spine and subsequently died. I was informed of her death whilst I was at school.

School turned out to be a 'safe haven' in terms of my mental health. I got to socialise, I was never bored and, towards the end of year 11, I became quite studious and actually left school with some qualifications. I am so pleased about the fact that my time wasn't wasted.

During my time at grammar school, I moved backwards and forwards from Mum's house to Dad's, the reason being that Mum would cry and tell me she was lonely. Even though I was a child, I thought that I could help. Mum always called me the 'adult' in the relationship. I always found this statement annoying, mainly due to the fact that she would read self help books and would often come out with 'psychobabble'. She would try to force me to read them. I had no concentration

TO SCHIZOPHRENIA AND BACK

and would get really irritated by her actions.

Eventually all of us ended up at Dad's, including Mum. I remember the police bringing her home after she had attempted to drive away from a pub and had crashed into a lamp post. It was years later that she found out that she had fractured one of her cervical vertebrae (neck) in the accident. The police visited pretty routinely in our household. Mum soon went back to living alone. I stayed at Dad's in the following years.

There was one time when I was in a road traffic accident and I was put in a position by my mother: to choose which home I was to go back to after being discharged from hospital following observations for a head injury and a fractured clavicle.

After the accident I began to yawn, I would yawn incessantly and I would get into trouble at school because of it. I find now that if I am not taking enough medicine, then I will start to yawn despite not being anxious or tired.

I chose Dad's house; the best thing I could have done.

Dad found a lovely woman, who became my step mum and they are very happy together to this day. They have retirement down to a fine art! I love

Annie Moon

them both very dearly.

Up until I moved again, at 15 to a new house with my step mum and my Dad, I would feel very spiritual by sneaking out of the house and walking around the streets in the middle of the night. On some occasions I would walk miles to see my friend, who would leave walkie talkies outside of her house so that I could wake her up to go wandering. Dad never said anything about this behaviour, despite the police stopping me and ringing my Dad up in the early hours of the morning.

Throughout my years living with my step mum I would be very paranoid. I would listen to the voices that I heard sitting at the top of the stairs. These voices would say nasty things about me, mainly that I was a waste of time, that I would not do well at school, all derogatory remarks.

In 1983 I attended a college of further education, I was 16 and I had no real idea of what I wanted to do for a living. My ambitions were leaning towards either being a physiotherapist, a lawyer, a police woman and my unattainable dream of becoming a doctor.

I met some lovely people at college, I had no problems socialising, however I was always a person of few words, I became quiet and I became a listener. I listened to one older girl who was discussing her hair loss caused by her vomiting.

TO SCHIZOPHRENIA AND BACK

She had anorexia and bulimia. I thought that this was a wonderful way of slimming down and subsequently developed bulimia myself.

I managed to lose over 28 pounds in 6 weeks on a calorie controlled diet and an exercise regime but once I'd lost the weight bulimia kicked in as a way of keeping it off. My studies suffered and I became very impulsive. I wanted to see the world!

Half way through my studies I asked a friend if she wanted to go on 'The Magic Bus', it would take us across Europe to Greece where I planned on 'island hopping'. I had saved money from some work that I did.

I worked in a shop selling 'nick knacks', tobacco, chocolate and stationary. I loved working there. In the evenings I would go to work as a barmaid in a public house. (I was under age at 17 to sell alcohol and they soon sussed me out when I hadn't a clue what I was doing. They were very nice about the whole thing, even though I had lied about my age.) They moved me onto collecting glasses before letting me go. My next job was in a service station, I found that the only way to get a job back then was to lie about my age so I told them that I was 18. I left when I was getting money taken out of my wages for things that shoplifters had stolen!

Annie Moon

I had over £200 pounds saved from money that I had earned working in a petrol station, in a shop and cleaning in my Dad's friend's pub. . . I bought my return bus tickets. I also got a special form from the post office. This would enable me to have treatment in another country. This was a positive thing to come out of Great Britain being part of the European Economic Community (EEC).

My friend took too long to make her mind up so I just went. She says now, 20 years later, that I just disappeared overnight after going into class and telling the tutor that I was going travelling and I would be back in a couple of months to sit my final exams!

ADVENTURES

I took a lovely air conditioned coach up to London, it even had a toilet on board and I was very impressed.

The magic bus from London to the ferry terminal was also lovely. Europe however was another matter!

The weather in Belgium was cold to say the least. It was the middle of the night and there was no connecting coach waiting for us. It was snowing, we were all travellers, some travelling alone, like

TO SCHIZOPHRENIA AND BACK

me, and some in couples. This atmosphere, although not very pleasant, turned into a good thing, it built up a kind of camaraderie which was to last throughout my trip.

There were a lot of Australian and New Zealand travellers. It was obvious that they were seasoned travellers; they took the situation all in their stride.

When the coach eventually turned up it was a rickety old Mercedes Benz that had seen better days. I suppose that for the price of the trip we should have been grateful even for a rickshaw. The coach's windows were so dirty that you couldn't see out of them. There were 2 drivers who were to take it in turn to drive across Europe to Athens in Greece. This turned out to be quite interesting and added lots of adventure and life experiences to my memory banks.

We travelled through Austria, passing steep mountains. It was very scary, as not only was it snowing, but you could see the driver falling in and out of sleep at the wheel. His co-driver was trying to get some sleep on the bus in a single seat. Things became nasty when the co-driver asked a passenger to give up his seat, so that the co-driver could lie down properly. There were punches exchanged and still the bus carried on precariously through the mountains.

Annie Moon

We did take break stops where we could freshen up, buy food and go to the toilet (as there was no toilet on this bus). I was able to say that I had been to a toilet in Belgium, Germany, Austria, Italy, Yugoslavia and Greece.

The toilet stop in Italy was not all it turned out to be. We went down some back streets away from the main road. When we arrived at the border to Yugoslavia not only did the driver fraudulently say that he wanted £5 off each of us all for visa's but the official on the border made a search of the bags and the coach (after the man who was punched earlier by the driver jumped out of the sliding window in the coach and ran to ask the guard if this visa story was true). The guards did a thorough search not only of all our bags but of the coach itself. The coach was to be turned back to Italy, leaving us all stranded at the border. The guards had found video players and a handgun. The drivers were to get rid of them before they were allowed to enter the country.

The Yugoslavian border facilities do lovely cheap spaghetti bolognaises! They did good business that day and luckily for us there were money exchanging facilities.

The coach wasn't too long in coming and we couldn't grumble because it was so cheap and luxurious compared to the previous toilet stops. The rest of the journey was unremarkable except for there being a great stench as we were all in the

TO SCHIZOPHRENIA AND BACK

same clothes that we set off in and also people had been smoking on the bus. We arrived in Athens about 3 days after getting on the coach in Belgium.

FIRST SYMPTOMS?

I travelled around Greece and I'm so glad that I did. I made many friends and was rarely alone, I even found a 'boyfriend' who I had a good 'snog' with.

I was homesick after about 4 weeks and after 6 weeks I decided to go home and sit my exams even though I had considered travelling to Israel to work on a Kibbutz.

I had met a Swedish girl who was bilingual; she could speak not only her own language and English, but French as well. We both went out socialising with 2 French men (purely platonic - on my part anyway). I loved to speak French at school and I asked my friend if she would only speak to me in French, which she did.

On the coach home I was hearing voices in French! When I thought somebody was speaking to me I would reply in French. I remember getting some funny looks, as the people whom I thought were speaking to me were actually from New Zealand and knew that I was English. I remember them saying disparaging remarks about me. I felt very self conscious and paranoid, I knew that I couldn't rely on my senses as I knew these people were from New Zealand and spoke English, so why would they speak French to me. I felt very stressed and embarrassed at times knowing that I was showing myself up. My coping mechanism then was to keep quiet and not say anything; my thoughts were my own and nobody could get in, or so I thought. Later in the years that followed, I thought that my thoughts could be read and I wasn't safe anywhere.

When I arrived back in Manchester, I was walking through Piccadilly gardens with my ruck-sack when a tramp approached me. I must have appeared to be homeless, having worn the same clothes for 4 days, also not having had a bath or shower in days. The tramp offered to give me 50 pence for a cup of tea. I was so spiritually touched by this gesture. A man, who had no home, was dirty and wearing tatty clothes was prepared to help others before himself. I thanked him and explained why I was looking so dishevelled.

During my travels I did not have any problems with weight issues.

Part of the 'new me' decided that I wanted to do a parachute jump for charity. I did this and enjoyed every minute of it. However I would think twice about doing such a 'stupid thing' now and I would

TO SCHIZOPHRENIA AND BACK

be a bag of nerves if one of my children said that they wanted to do a parachute jump.

I have felt that 'today would be a good day to die' on a few occasions, one being on the back of my brother 'Nobby's' motorbike when he was travelling at over a 100 miles per hour whilst doing a 'wheelie', one occasion being my parachute jump and one time being when I was on the infamous 'Big One' roller coaster ride at Blackpool.

On those occasions when I was not scared of dying, the feelings were like the feelings I get when I feel in tune with God. I feel that he is communicating with me through television programmes, notices in shop windows, signs in the pavements and through electricity waves sent through the high tension cables on pylons, especially when the rain hits them.

After returning home I went back to college and sat my exams, all but one of them. During my last months at college, I got a job, (again after telling fibs about my age). I was almost 18 years old. The job was in an old people's home and I thought that I would try to become a nurse after this experience, even though I was under a great deal of stress at the home. The matron was always in the office and there were lots of residents to get up and lots of beds to make and so little time to do it. With this stress my eating disorder reared its ugly head.

The bulimia became an unpleasant part of my life; it became more of a coping strategy rather than a weight matter. I did approach my doctor about it when I was so distressed that I felt suicidal. I will talk about this later.

TO SCHIZOPHRENIA AND BACK

CHAPTER THREE

NURSE TRAINING

I was eighteen whilst I was working as a carer in an 'old peoples' home'. I decided to apply to train as a nurse. This was something that I definitely would not have considered when I was younger, the reason being that I had seen how hard my step mum worked (she was a trained nurse) on the care of the elderly wards. I sometimes went in to help out at the hospital at night time.

I sent my application form in on the Monday; by the Thursday I received a phone call, asking me to attend an interview the next day (Friday). I attended my interview on the Friday; that same day I had a medical and, due to a cancelled place in the school of nursing's intake, I was offered a place practically straight away.

I was immature emotionally because I had not had the role models to emulate during my childhood. I was also scarred due to some of the emotional abuse from my birth mother. I found it very difficult not to say what I was thinking about somebody out loud. I was unreservedly honest to my detriment. On one occasion, a Nursing Sister on a ward said to me that unless this particular patient came to the dining table she would not get fed. The patient asked for my help and I just

Annie Moon

relayed word for word what the Sister had said! Needless to say, this lady was particularly upset. So was the Sister and I 'copped for it'.

I had no social skills to speak of. Throughout my younger years I had very little adult stimulation, in the way of conversation or help in coping with stressful situations. My step mum provided that in my late teens but I had a lot of catching up to do to make up for the years of 'social isolation'.

It was around this time, whilst I was still living with my step mum and Dad, that I was becoming increasingly paranoid. I constantly thought that they were discussing me with their friends in a very negative way. I would hear things, which I now believe were auditory hallucinations, calling me bad and unworthy of any love. I 'heard' that I would 'amount to nothing'.

What resulted from this paranoia was a physical attack by me towards my step mum. I truly am sorry for that to this day.

There were many occasions when I felt stressed, one occasion being when a patient died of cancer. This particular patient had been ill for a long time and was also very old (in his 90's). Subsequently the patient had lost a lot of weight and he had also been suffering with mouth ulcers. The reason for my stress was that this patient had died and needed 'laying out'. In those days students were left to 'get on with it'. Not long after the patient

TO SCHIZOPHRENIA AND BACK

had died there was a disciplinary procedure in progress. I had put the patient's false teeth in the property bag because they would not fit into the patient's mouth. I can understand how distressing that must have been, for the relative to find, but I must say this; there are a lot of unnecessary complaints which take nurses away from their patients and leave them 'traumatised'. I found over the years that those relatives who have been absent in the lives of their loved ones are often the ones to be making the most complaints; it's as if they feel that they need to be making themselves useful, albeit in an unconstructive way. I must say, however,- that there are 'goings on' that need to be addressed for health, safety and human decency.

I feel that doing my nurse training has turned me into a worldly person; seeing life and death situations. I feel that I have learned a lot about human nature.

After 1 year of nursing study I fell in love and married my husband, whom I will talk about in the next chapter.

I was fortunate enough to get a staff nurse job on regular night duty on a medical ward. I really enjoyed this work and seemed to get along with most of the staff.

Annie Moon

Things started to fall apart when I was trying for my second son. I had a very early miscarriage- a home pregnancy test kit came up positive and my period was late, however a few days later I bled. The family doctor said that a high percentage of foetuses abort very early on, usually due to abnormalities, so I was not unduly affected when it was explained to me in that way.

I started having trouble sleeping. My neighbour was a D.I.Y. enthusiast and their teenage children would play loud music during the day, as mine do now!

After my second son was born it became even harder to sleep as I seemed to work a lot of weekends and my husband was at home looking after the children who were noisy. It never crossed my mind to ask for some sleeping tablets- I'm sure that my doctor wouldn't have given them to me anyway! With hindsight, I could have stopped at my Dad's house to sleep, but I felt that it was my home and I should be there. I didn't blame anybody as night duty was my choice, but at the time I couldn't see a way out of the extreme, sickly tiredness that I was feeling (I was breastfeeding my younger son also- I would often go home during my break and feed him).

I don't know how it came about, but I think my clairvoyant phase started after a night of ghost stories. One night I went to a secluded area of a very old ward, it was dark and eerie. I sensed a

TO SCHIZOPHRENIA AND BACK

really bad presence and became quite afraid- I realise now that I am no more a clairvoyant than a telephone poll (although this feeling is transient depending on how well I am!)

I was asked on a couple of occasions by friends to go with them to a clairvoyant's house and then to a spiritualist church. When I had my readings done, the clairvoyants (I call them soothsayers- this is because my Mum would avidly read the Bible in her 'born again Christian' phase and would try to force me to read it whilst quoting out of it and she said that in the Bible 'soothsayers' are evil.) would not predict my future but would tell me that I had the 'Gift' and try to show me some of the ways to use it.

I tried reading peoples' jewellery at work on our breaks. People kept coming back for more and said that my readings were accurate! This really spooked me and I began seeing spirits. I moved on to tarot cards and began reading my own; apparently according to clairvoyants this is something that you must never do. Even my boss had hers read a few times during breaks. This 'hocus pocus' never affected my work until I became troubled by voices and visions telling me to go to the moors in the middle of winter and in the middle of the night to await death- at this point I couldn't even think about work and I took sick leave.

Annie Moon

The level of understanding during this bout of illness was a totally different experience from that I had had when I was pregnant. The management were very understanding and accommodating and the support that I got from colleagues was memorable to say the least. They would visit me in hospital and at home and people would telephone asking how I was- however one person did telephone for selfish reasons and that was to ask me how much money I was getting on the sick, because she was contemplating sick leave herself!

Prior to my first full blown breakdown, I had a 'busy mind'. I wanted to undertake lots of nursing courses and got frustrated when I seemingly received little support, despite me paying for them myself and not through work. I also tried to get into the police force and got right the way through lots of tests, e.g. observation and physical tests but failed miserably on the psychometric testing- fancy that! In hindsight, I was as mad as they come!

I believed I was the victim of a management bully at work and was so paranoid about being persecuted that I even taped our phone conversations! When a psychiatrist asked me if she said anything on the tapes to prove this bullying I said 'no' which was true; I was just paranoid and deluded!

After my first diagnosed episode of schizophrenia,

TO SCHIZOPHRENIA AND BACK

I was given lots of help to return to work. They reduced my hours and put me on days. This all seems very helpful; however it was totally the opposite. I had no childcare, I hadn't worked on days for a number of years and I was worried about how it would affect my pay, after all we did have a mortgage to pay. I was also unable to take medication and stay awake for any workable length of time.

I did try days, everybody was helpful but I felt that I had to stop my medication to function properly and to be able to be alert at work. The stopping of medication meant that my symptoms returned and so I had to go back on sick leave.

CHAPTER FOUR

FAMILY LIFE
MY MARRIAGE

First of all I dedicate this book to my husband and children who have given me something to live for when times have gotten really bad.

I have been married for nearly 21 years to a wonderful man whose nickname is 'Todd'. He was 23 and I was eighteen when we met.

I met Todd whilst I was out at a pub, with a friend from college. I prided myself on being able to go out socialising on a pittance of 50 pence. I would make one orange juice and water last me all night.

I really fancied Todd from the first moment I laid eyes on him. He had lovely dark hair and he was in the Royal Air Force. He also was very sociable and had a big group of friends with whom he hung around.

I mentioned that I liked him to my friend. She said that the feeling was mutual but that he had a girlfriend already. I said that I would not date somebody who already had a partner.

Not long after our first meeting and after a few relayed messages, Todd rang me up. He had left the Air Force and was single. He asked me out for a drink but insisted that I buy my own as he

TO SCHIZOPHRENIA AND BACK

was currently looking for work!

Taking a pride in being 'thrifty' myself I welcomed the honesty and a little part of me thought that he was a man after my own heart!

We dated for 4 months without having sex. It was at a party that I explained that I would love to have sex with him but for the fact that I was not on any form of contraception. I said that if he wanted to have sex, then he would have to go to the family planning clinic with me. He went with me and that was that sorted out!

Todd asked me to marry him whilst he was quite drunk one night over a Christmas period. I accepted but I asked him the next morning if he remembered the proposal and he did. I was only eighteen at the time, he was twenty three.

I lived in a friend's house after being thrown out of the family home after my assault on my step-mum. This friend Rob was to be the best man at our wedding. He was a life long friend of Todd's. He was in the army and he let me stop while he was away at work. Thank you, Rob; I'm forever in your debt- if it wasn't for this help I couldn't have carried on nursing without a place to live.

I then moved onto sharing a flat with a woman who had outlived three husbands! I didn't stop there for too long!

It was not long before Todd and I found and bought our first home together. That was in April. We got married that August. The budget was very tight- however it's the best wedding that I've ever been to!

After 2 years of studying we planned our first child and I caught straight away.

I was entitled to maternity leave towards the end of the pregnancy. During the pregnancy I was seen as somebody who needed 'carrying'. There is a lot of bullying in a hospital staffed mainly by females. Life as a pregnant student nurse was very stressful. When I was lifting patients I was, as the nurses would say, 'putting my baby at risk'. When I wasn't lifting, i.e. doing other essential jobs, like checking blood observations, temperatures, pulses and blood pressures, I was seen as a burden.

When I was a student nurse, I found nights very difficult to cope with. I would go to bed at 8am and not wake up until 8pm. I felt overstretched, I wasn't coping very well and I needed a rest. It was not unusual for me to be there at the last minute for a night shift!

Thanks to my understanding doctor realising how distressed I was getting due to what seemed to me to be the silent bullying, I was able to take the

TO SCHIZOPHRENIA AND BACK

last few months off work.

It was while I was pregnant that my unborn baby took precedence. My eating problems went away; I exercised and ate all the right nutrients in my food. I have never smoked and I did not take any alcohol.

My first son was born weighing 7lb 4oz. He was born healthy with a mild birth defect which was rectified by a specialist plastic surgeon; it is thanks to him that my son has no lasting damage.

Refreshed from my maternity leave and nice and slim as a result of breast feeding, a good diet and plenty of exercise, I was ready to face the world. I would spend hours walking our dog in the local park whilst pushing the buggy or having No 1 son in a harness strapped to me. This period of my life was the happiest. When I smell certain things even today I recognise them from these times and I feel an overwhelming sense of peace, happiness and warmth washing over me.

I found it extremely pleasurable to nurse with my new outlook on life. My studying capabilities were phenomenal. I breezed through the rest of my training only taking a few days off when my son was attacked by our Doberman bitch.

I was in our home, a lovely refurbished terraced

Annie Moon

house; I was sat on the floor revising for nursing exams when my son was walking around the furniture. My son was 14 months old. The bitch was like a child to us, she was 8 years old, and she was laid on the settee when my son touched her paw. The bitch was called Duchess; we had treated her like a child. She used to sleep on our bed with us, she was a beautiful creature. When No 1 son was born, she used to walk by the side of the buggy, but her behaviour started to change. I would never leave my son alone in the same room, I would not let her near him whilst I was holding him; in effect I had pushed her out of the picture. Duchess began taking abnormal notice of motorbikes going past and where previously she walked unleashed by the side of the buggy, she then changed to wanting to chase motorbikes. In hindsight she was suffering from stress and probably felt rejected. Duchess picked my son up by his head using her teeth, one jaw in his chin and the other on top of his head, like a vice. I was right next to them. I jumped up and punched her until she let go.

My son was bleeding and crying, I was not on the telephone and my neighbours were out, so I went to a betting shop with him across the street from our house.

As I walked into the shop the patrons who filled the shop all stood back against the walls as I shouted for help in getting an ambulance. After only seconds one man, whom to this day I have

TO SCHIZOPHRENIA AND BACK

yet to thank properly, stood forwards and said, 'I'll take you to the hospital love'.

At the hospital they did skull x-rays which needed reporting on by a consultant as it was suspected that my son had a fractured skull. He has a permanent scar on his lip which is not noticeable 17 years later and he has a tiny area on his skull that has no hair. He loves dogs and is constantly on at me for one.

Duchess was put to sleep in our home on the next day and when I am not particularly well I often feel her and sense that she is still with us; on occasion I have seen her, especially when I am feeling 'liquidy and spiritual'.

I often get prodromal symptoms which often begin with 'feeling liquidy'. I would describe this as a feeling of floating around people and looking in on society from a spiritual stance. I feel that I am on the outside looking in and that I am not part of the human race. I often wonder if I have been sent to Earth to fulfil a mission, I often wonder if I am one of God's helpers as I feel so spiritual at the time.

At this particular house I often thought that I could see an old guard from the time of Oliver Cromwell. Was this an hallucination?

We moved not long after that incident and round

about the same time my mother in law died. My mother in law was a character. She was very ill with cancer and I spent some time with her helping her to wash and I also gave her emotional support as she knew that she was dying.

I often feel that I can see dead people as spirits; I also feel a presence and am convinced that they are speaking to me or can read my mind and plant thoughts in my head.

We decided to move house shortly after this episode in our lives.

My new house had everything that I had wished for, a garden, patio doors, an oven and hob and was lovely and bright.

At the age of 21, I had my own home, a marriage, a baby and I'd just qualified and got a part time job as a registered nurse. Things couldn't have been better.

I loved my job as a nurse. I worked 30 hours a week over 3 nights. Not long after qualifying I was able to take charge of the ward.

Once I was able to qualify for maternity leave again we planned our next baby. It took 12 months before I conceived. I did have what I consider to be a very early miscarriage a few months after trying for a baby. My doctor said that if it wasn't for these extremely accurate over the

TO SCHIZOPHRENIA AND BACK

counter testing kits most people would think that they'd had a late period. This was said in a sensitive way, which helped, as he explained that a lot of foetuses are aborted naturally, early on. Work again was very stressful at this time. The 'caring profession' was not very caring when it came to pregnancy.

I became pregnant as planned and we had another healthy 7lb 12oz baby boy. I was to breastfeed my youngest son for 2 1/2 years. It was the best thing for my son but not for my health. I would go home during my break on my night shift to give him milk. I would also feed him whilst I should have been sleeping and on my days/nights off I would not get a decent night sleep, because he didn't sleep through a full night.

I've calculated that I didn't get a full night's sleep for fourteen years as there was a problem with bed wetting with the children for a long time (something I think runs in the family with boys, as I remember one of my brothers having the same problem) so I would get up and toilet the boys, or if I was too late the youngest would get into bed with us; I was so tired!! Looking back with hindsight there was a lot I could have done. I could have asked for help from the enuresis nurse, but I didn't agree with using bed wetting alarms as I thought that this would make the youngest a nervous wreck! I could have retrained the habit of him

Annie Moon

getting into bed with us, as I have since seen programmes on television teaching you how to do this. This would have been invaluable help as a young working mum. The television programmes came too late for me!

Anyway they've turned out O.K. and don't have any problems sleeping now!

Moving on to the schizophrenia, it really took hold when number two son was about eighteen months old. I was still breastfeeding him and nipping home in the night to do so, on my breaks from nursing. I was getting more and more paranoid, especially concerning matters involving my birth mum. She would treat the children differently, by taking one out and not the other. She was a bit odd herself and when challenged about her behaviour towards No 2 son, she said 'I had an abortion because I couldn't look after any more children'. I told her that she was not welcome in our house if treating my children differently. Todd thought it was because of his name as it is Scandinavian and religion based. My birth mum was very odd when it came to religion, she had been a born again Christian for a while, constantly pushing her Bible in my face and quoting passages whilst recommending that I read some. When she wasn't thrusting the Bible on to me she was encouraging me to read Alcoholics Anonymous' 12 Steps as she was a recovering alcoholic.

TO SCHIZOPHRENIA AND BACK

I believe strongly in Christianity; however I don't go to church except on special occasions; yet I always thank God for my life with my children and family and I always ask for guidance should circumstances be trying. I always say, 'Dear God, I know that you have plans for me, please guide me in the right direction'.

My reason for not going is that I just cry when I have gone in the past to worship! I don't know what all that is about!

And hey, things usually work out! I also feel that there are lots of opportunities in life and we have lots of choices to make. I can understand how someone with any mental illness can turn to street drugs, but no-one can force you unless you are in exceptional circumstances. You must make up your own mind through choices and have an enlightened perspective on things. One wise CPN said to me never make decisions when you are angry. This was excellent advice and has saved me from many a potential problem.

Whilst at work I felt as though I was being stifled, I wanted to do courses; I was running too fast with my plans. I did do courses but these, with lack of sleep, work and breastfeeding all took their toll. I became extremely paranoid as discussed in chapter three.

Annie Moon

The only input from family at this time was the occasional help from my Dad and step mum. They had their lives to live and they had two big Dobermans living with them. I remember at one Christmas meal they did for us, my step sister's daughter was coming back to the dining room from the toilet, and she just made it into the dining room as Duke snapped his jaws at her. Dad said that it 'was only a love bite'; something that still haunts me now!

When I had to have time off from nursing on sick leave, I still managed to get the children to heir activities, school, playgroup etc.

I was so exhausted from being unable to sleep properly that I would often go home and sleep for a couple of hours in a chair. I bought myself a wind up alarm clock so that I would be woken up in time to pick number two son up from playgroup. On a couple of occasions I had to telephone my step mum, who then kindly picked him up and gave him some dinner, his favourite being home made pizza and chips.

During most of my hospital admissions I was very selective over visitors. During the first admission I was visited very regularly by my husband and the children, as well as by friends from work, who were extremely supportive. I remember asking Mark, one of my dearest friends, where he was going to on holiday- he said that I had asked the same question several times and did ask me if I

TO SCHIZOPHRENIA AND BACK

was doing a 'Spike Milligan' for a bit of time off work! We laugh about this now.

I was too ashamed to see my Dad and step mum, my birth mum had said that I was attention seeking and quite honestly I felt as though I was in a freak show with people coming to see how dysfunctional I had become.

My Dad and step mum were invited to write a letter for this book, addressing the readers, this is what they wrote:-

When Annie first showed signs of stress and mood swings, we didn't really worry too much, putting it down to mixing full time work as a staff nurse with bringing up a young family, but as time went on and she suffered set back after set back, we became both worried and concerned, mainly for Annie herself, but also for Todd, her husband, and the boys, who were only young at the time.

For a long time we were both confused and hurt by her withdrawal during her bad times. When she had good days and weeks we were hopeful of a full recovery.

As we gained more understanding of the management and medication of her illness, we became so very proud of her ability to cope and of her many achievements.

Annie Moon

Words of hindrance to recovery that I have had:

You are attention seeking (Birth mother)
There's nothing wrong with you (Aunty who sees me every few years)
'You don't need medication' (step mum- in the early days and   I said this to myself on many occasions when the medication was working and making me feel a lot better).
'You've put on some weight' (colleagues and a CPN).
'You're just doing it for a free bus pass' (Aunty who I've seen less than 10 times in my life; I think this was meant jokingly as she's normally a very caring person).
'You just want benefit payments' (various people).

Words that have spurred me on:-
'You are not expected to work again' (CPN)
'What do you want to give up you're benefits for?' (Husband)
'Why are you doing a paper round, that's a young person's job?' (This was said by a CPN, when I ended up managing my children's paper rounds; I was amazed that my efforts to get back to normality were commented on like this).
'Don't be a victim', (words from my sister who doesn't know me!)

My friend Brenda often boosted my self esteem when I was sad. She'd send me cards when

TO SCHIZOPHRENIA AND BACK

she'd not heard from me or when I wasn't answering the telephone.

She sent me a lovely fridge magnet saying 'Mothers are Angels in training'. This meant so much to me, as I had a personal prejudice against myself and my own illness and I believed that people thought that I shouldn't be looking after my children, when I know that I've done a pretty good job despite my obstacles.

When asked if she would like to write for this book Brenda wrote the following:-

When Annie told me that she was writing a book on her experience of schizophrenia, I wasn't at all surprised; she has consistently surprised me so I think that I've sort of developed an 'expect the unexpected' outlook and consider all her projects calmly.

I don't like to think of her experiences as a schizophrenic because I know the breezy, loveable infectious, giggly person whom I care for has experienced some harrowing emotions. When she told me that she thought child remains were buried under her floor I felt inadequate to support her; she never complains about such thoughts in a way that you would find acceptable. She is matter of fact and direct. I can never recall her expanding on any of her distressing thoughts; she only elaborates on the ones that upset people the least, such as setting up a brothel; at one time I thought she was half joking and we don't mind talking about sex- we discussed specialities, preferences and dislikes!!! It was only when she'd told me she'd looked for premises that I realised that her commitment to the idea was real.

In contrast to the harrowing emotions some of Annie's visions have been hilarious. I think sex again was the motive behind her police application, I know that she likes the uniform. Strangely enough she has a fondness for the force and always talks of their professionalism when they've recovered her from the moors; I don't know if it's a testimony to the genuine nature of police officers or Annie's tendency to mainly talk about the more humorous side of schizophrenia, because she does see one and we often discuss what is normal. We share the view that most people go 'undiagnosed' or don't acknowledge their individuality. I am a recovered alcoholic and I hope this won't affect peoples' judgment on my views of Annie; if anything the reverse, as at the height of my suicidal tendencies, fuelled by drink, I remember Annie's support and encouragement; I also remember thinking she's able to support me while she's so ill herself.

I hope I'm not giving a false impression of Annie's coping skills; I know the lows must have been extremely low and there is a lot I feel that she must have kept from me, not out of

TO SCHIZOPHRENIA AND BACK

embarrassment or inhibition but out of choice. Annie has had numerous stays on the psychiatric unit and I know her marriage has been under strain from situations and just from life, but when I think of Annie I think of fun. She is near to completing her social work course, has a close family with her husband and two sons and I feel that she has been on what I can only describe as a non stop, hectic, sometimes adrenaline fuelled journey. While the lows have been so low, the highs have been just that. Annie was one of only two people able to come to my 40th and whilst I fretted and thought it's a non event already, Annie brought the atmosphere with her; she made it such a lovely time. I can't remember who had the candy floss pink wig, but Annie turned it into a party piece with everyone trying it on. It sounds corny but she made my 40th celebrations.

I feel sad often that Annie has had to experience anything of schizophrenia, not sad in a sentimental way, but in a reflective way. I think her optimism, love of life and mischievousness has made her a survivor, not bitter, just again matter of fact. When she told me of complaining to her consultant that the medication was affecting her sex life, I laughed but thought she's never given much 'complaining time' to the other side-effects of her medication, she will mention them briefly, but not at length. I'm very proud of Annie, she has achieved so much, she has numerous

Annie Moon

friends not because of her hospital admissions and professional courses, although they must have widened her field of contact, but because she has, despite a life affecting condition (for her family also) remained sunny, a breath of fresh air at times, with a reserve of compassion for others that is inspiring. I know her book will help others and it might at times be distressing to read but, although I haven't yet read her work, I'm sure it will show her humour, resilience and positive outlook on her view of being a schizophrenic; then for Annie that will be another achievement in dispelling negative views, fuelling optimism, challenging convention and simply sharing her life's experiences.

Another present off Brenda was a picture frame whose contents said 'Believe in yourself'. :-

'I know you have within you
everything you need,
many special qualities
to help you to succeed.
I just wanted you to know
that I believe in you,
and hope that you
will always
believe in yourself too.
(Heartwarmers Frame WPL London. U.K.)

It is helpful to have simple poetry of this sort around, I have another one from:-

TO SCHIZOPHRENIA AND BACK

M&S Co-operative Society-
The Hallmark of Value-
Rule 17

<u>It Can Be Done</u>

Somebody said that it couldn't be done
But he, with a chuckle replied
That maybe it couldn't but he would be one
Who wouldn't say so till he tried.

So he buckled right in, with a trace of a grin
On his face, if he worried, he hid it;
He started to sing as he tackled the thing
That couldn't be done, and he did it.

Somebody scoffed, 'Oh you'll never do that
At least no one ever has done it,'
But he took off his coat and he took off his hat
And the first thing he knew he'd begun it.
There are thousands to tell you it cannot be done;
There are thousands to prophesy failure;
There are thousands to point out to you one by one
The dangers that wait to assail you.

But just buckle right in with a bit of a grin,
Throw off your coat and go to it:
Just start to sing as you tackle the thing
That cannot be done, and you'll do it.

Annie Moon

Some of the things that people said were on the whole probably well meant. I however decided to prove a point and that is that I am not going to be seen and be written off as a social misfit who shuffles around psychiatric wards in between bouts of potential violence.

If I am to get attention it will be for my achievements!
I will not be seen as a victim- I am a fighter!
I want to come off benefits, I see work as a privilege or else why would they let prisoners have jobs for good behaviour!

I have been indignant at some of the comments which have made me work even harder to break the mould!

Now I will get off my soap box!

I had never thought of how many children I wanted to have when I was younger. Todd was the one to bring the subject up after we had been married for about a year. He very nauseatingly said one night in bed 'wouldn't it be nice to hear the pitter patter of tiny feet?'

I agreed, despite me being half way through my full time nursing course. However it was the most worthwhile thing that I have ever undertaken. I have always thought that children are a gift from

TO SCHIZOPHRENIA AND BACK

God and are so precious. We went on to have number one son then number two son a few years later.

The problem came when I wanted a third child. Todd said that he wanted to be 'more selfish' and spend some of his money and time on himself.

I yearned for a third child for a few years and often felt that I could have quite easily tricked Todd into impregnating me, however I felt that another child would need the full attention and affection from their father and this would always be affected if they were born out of deceit.

When I became quite ill, I used to think that I might be pregnant as the medication often made my periods irregular or absent altogether, this with the hope of a child and the weight gain from medication made me put two and two together and come up with 109!

I began questioning my right to have more children when I had been diagnosed with schizophrenia. I thought that if I did have more children then they would be put on the child protection register. I really valued my role as a mother, but in the back of my mind I was always imagining what the general public would think.

I approached Todd about having a vasectomy, he

agreed and that was that. I did say to him in all honesty, that if he didn't want any more children it should be he who has the 'snip'; I on the other hand should keep my options open should I find a new partner.

As the years have gone on, I'm glad we stopped when we did, as we have more time to do the things we couldn't do when the children were younger. The stress of having older children is a different kind of stress to that of when they were younger. Younger children need protecting from danger; older children not only need this in a different way, but you have to step back and advise from a distance, in effect, begin to 'let go'.

When the children were young and I was ill, one thing that was very lacking was the help available for child care whilst I went to the psychiatric day hospital. We were told that, because the children were not 'children in need' and Todd worked, nobody could help. I have brought this need for crèche facilities up at users' forums for the attention of managers. I have never followed this up as my need for childcare and day hospital services has not been necessary in recent years.

Contact with family members only happens when I am well, as does contact with friends. I tend to withdraw from the outside world and become totally immersed in my thoughts which very often are paranoid in nature. I stop answering the telephone and I have even been known to hide

TO SCHIZOPHRENIA AND BACK

from people whom I have seen or thought that I have seen in the street or on the moors (my world in the sky).

My friends have been very supportive. We often go for walks or to the pictures or out for lunch when I am well. I remember asking Mark if we could go to the theme park for the white knuckle rides- he took me when I was on a great deal of medication and I thoroughly enjoyed the thrills, again I would think that 'this is a good day to die!'

When in hospital one time Todd took the lads on holiday- without me! They went abroad to Majorca, a Spanish island. I should have gone but a great deal of anxiety and depression overtook me and I ended up back in hospital. This was in the very early days. My problem was post psychotic depression- something I am an expert in handling these days.

When I felt better after about a week, I managed to get myself a plane ticket and found my way to the hotel. Todd didn't speak to me for a whole day. One of the sunbathers next to the hotel pool said that they had thought that he was a single dad and had thought of befriending him. I was sad at this and cried and cried silently beneath my sunglasses.

There were issues around sex, my libido and my

Annie Moon

ability to orgasm. This was all due to medication and with good communication with my consultant the medications were adjusted or changed to meet my needs. One of the worst offenders was an anti-depressant drug, which I came off altogether. I will discuss more about how I personally 'nipped' depression in the 'bud', without the need for me to take ante-depressants in chapter seven, which is about my rehabilitation.

When my eldest brother died after years of self abuse and neglect as a result of drug and alcohol addiction; it was not a great shock. He was only forty; sometimes I wonder if I myself will see forty during the bad times.

Steven was a very kind unassuming man who was badly let down during his upbringing. He lived with my Dad during all of his childhood. My birth mum moved us all out of the house whilst he was at school and he didn't know until he got home that his mother and siblings had left him and my dad.

I think that my Dad tried his best; he was a hard worker and a hard player, in the sense that he liked a drink at the pub.

Steven came to my house a few months before he died; he was homeless. He said that a man had died in the back yard of the house where he was living. The other housemates brought him into the kitchen and rifled through his pockets- apparently

TO SCHIZOPHRENIA AND BACK

the police were very unhappy about this to say the least!

Steven also told me about a time when he stole a single shoe from outside of a shoe shop. He was arrested for this and in his defence he replied that he had stolen it for his one legged friend- the magistrate told him not to be so facetious! The story was actually very true, he did have a one legged friend.

Steven often had a humorous way with words.

He was invited to stay until I could help him the next day at housing aid. He was jaundiced and emaciated. My CPN at the time tried very hard to get him some kind of help but she met with resistance trying to contact people due to confidentiality.

The next day, Steven and I went to get him registered at a doctor's surgery and we then went on to housing aid. They wanted to put him in a hostel for men. I explained that he was trying to come off drugs and alcohol and that this would only compound the problem. They listened to us and Steven was invited to a hostel where he would be supported to get and keep clean.

The room was lovely and clean and there was a kitchenette in another part of the room. I bought

Annie Moon

him some groceries and essentials such as towels, soap etc. I felt cold when he complained to me that he would have to use some of his benefit to cover the cost of staying there, as the benefits people would only pay so much. I thought, and was a bit angry, that he was getting help and he didn't appreciate it. Later he very nicely went on to tell me that my brother had said that I was a carbon copy of my birth mother. I wasn't upset about this analogy, however I was annoyed. He must have realised that this would offend me; needless to say the next time I saw him was at the mortuary. I can honestly say that I couldn't have helped more than I did.

At Steven's funeral there was an obvious divide. All siblings were separated by an invisible distain for each other.

Dad broke down and cried, something that I'd never seen him do before.

I felt that I didn't really know anything about him, so I decided to ask around. I asked his brother what things were like as children and adolescents. Things were clarified, stories were validated and things were put straight- I felt better, more grounded in myself by having knowledge. I would recommend speaking to family members if possible about how things were in the past- maybe then it can be understood where people are coming from. Communication should not be left until there's a death to deal with. A lot of healing can be done if we are honest with each

TO SCHIZOPHRENIA AND BACK

other.

A few years ago, my dad who is heading for seventy years old, asked me to sit and have a chat with him one night. Todd, the boys and I were all stopping in their seaside bungalow where they have retired to. Just Dad and I were up late one night having a drink and Dad, out of the blue, said "Ann tell me about your life and your friends". I nearly fell off the chair! I had never experienced this before. Dad was not one for talking to us let alone talking about feelings. As I began talking, Dad said that I mustn't be so hard on people. I commented on some things that people did that I didn't like and spoke of how I will not embrace people who were in any way mean to me. Dad went on to apologise for my childhood- something that I had not discussed ever with him. As far as I am concerned, despite my Dads liking for the pub, he did a good job. I was very humbled by his apology- something that I have done with my own children, apologised to them. I think that when well meant, this can mend a lot of bridges.

Mental health problems do not run in Dad's side of the family. However on my birth mother's side, her mum, my maternal grandma, had bipolar disorder; I wonder now if she actually had schizophrenia herself. I thought the world of 'Nana'. We often wrote many letters to each other and I often went to stay with her during the holidays as she lived at the seaside. I am sad that I never went to pay my respects at her funeral due to my fragile mental state at the time. I did send a wreath and was anxious that they spelt Nana wrong. When I am 'not myself' I sometimes 'see' my Nana and we communicate very often 'telepathically'; all symptoms of the schizophrenia but when this happens it is very hard not to think that I am a clairvoyant.

My birth mum suffered a lot with depression and alcohol abuse when I was younger. I don't know how she is doing now as I keep my distance in a self protective way, to maintain my sanity.

I remember her becoming very agitated about some words from a song that I had written down when I was about eleven years old. I became very fearful of her and thought that she was going to 'batter' me. That's the funny thing about my childhood with my mother; I can't remember her ever hitting me like she did the others. I felt a lot of fear towards her; I had good cause as I had seen what she was capable of physically when I had seen her abuse my siblings.

I know that my birth mum had a lot of input from psychiatrists and social workers etc. She never did say what was wrong with her, only that she was an alcoholic.

TO SCHIZOPHRENIA AND BACK

I remember her taking an overdose and writing on her wallpaper just above her bed- I can't remember what she had written.

One time she messed around with a ouija board. She wrote down on a piece of paper jumbled up words and pinned them to the chimney breast for weeks.

When I was older and Todd and I stopped at her house overnight, on a sofa bed downstairs, she came down during the night, fumbled about in the kitchen, it sounded like her going into the cutlery drawer and we heard her say that she was going to stab us.

I also had to warn Todd about the possibility of her making a pass at him as she had done previously with my sister's boyfriend.

On the subject of family history of mental illness, again on my mum's side of the family, a young cousin also has schizophrenia.

During periods of ill health I would often wander onto the moors to meet with God and to get a bit of peace with the spirits in the open air thereby protecting my children??? Total nonsense when I am thinking straight.

Annie Moon

Many a time the police would be called and on a couple of occasions the police helicopter has been deployed. I say this in a very ashamed manner, although some would say I *was* ill at the time. I have a friend who says that she would like a helicopter to come and rescue her!!

I have had conversations with Todd about what goes on at home when I am not myself having been admitted to the psychiatric unit. He said that when I get reported as missing, the police search every closet, shed and garage on our property to make sure that he hasn't 'done away' with me. Todd has also said that in the early days he'd 'wished that I had died on the moors'. This comment broke my heart. We worked through this and my thoughts on this are that it's ok to speak and be open and honest. Sometimes the truth hurts. It took a while for me not to bring up this comment every time I was ill.

Even now he can't help himself with little quips such as 'what planet are you on', or 'is there anybody in there?'

Recently we watched a programme about a serial killer who had a personality disorder. She was in Rampton Mental Hospital. This is a secure unit. When I asked Todd where it was, he offered to drop me off there the next time we pass it!

Normally these things wash over me and I take them as black humour. However if I am feeling

TO SCHIZOPHRENIA AND BACK

agitated I don't hesitate in speaking my mind in a very civilised, articulate way. On a couple of occasions I have explained that his words are akin to goading an alcoholic about their problem, that it's cruel and should not be done- basically it's not funny.

I have explained to Todd that if he doesn't like me then he should feel free to find somewhere else to live. I have even drawn up a financial plan for him at these times!

Of course 99% of the time we get along just fine. Todd wrote the following for the book:-

Life with someone you love who as a mental illness can best be summed up in a couple of clichés, the first one being "it's like a box of chocolates, you never know what you'll get"; I mean this in so much as you go to sleep with everything ok, then the next morning the person is totally changed in mood and behaviour. The other cliché is "life is a rollercoaster, full of highs and lows" only in this case you will not always be able to see ahead and know what's coming.

The first symptoms of Annie's mental illness were not, to me, an actual sign of mental problems. As I had never come across this before, I considered it more to be a breaking down in our relationship. The difficulty with this was that I could not see why

Annie Moon

this was happening and as a consequence became a bit distant myself while I was trying to understand what was happening and how best to deal with it. The first time I realised it was more than just a relationship problem is still very vivid in my mind as I will now explain.

I had always, even since before we were first married, gone out most Friday nights with a group of old mates, nothing more than a chance to drink beer and put the world right as we see it. This particular night was one of the odd occasions when I was staying in, it was late autumn and cold, Annie was again being uncommunicative and very distant. She put the children to bed by about 9pm, then suddenly announced she was going out for a drive. I said nothing and just assumed that this was it, "the end", and she was off to meet someone. I waited in watching the TV but not really aware of what I was watching, just twisting scenarios of what action to take constantly around in my head. Eventually about midnight I took myself to bed but hardly slept, I heard Annie come in around 6am and immediately asked where she had been. I got what by now was a fairly typical response, "none of your business" and she then just went up to bed. That morning, whilst making the kids' breakfast and generally mulling about the house, I noticed in her handbag, on the dining table, a small bread knife and then spotted a diary type booklet. Obviously I had to read this to get an insight into what was going on. I had two reactions to what I read: first relief that it

TO SCHIZOPHRENIA AND BACK

wasn't an affair, then shock as to what can only be described as weird rambling. I was able to spot immediately that this was a sign of what looked like the beginning of a major breakdown and that medical help was needed.

I managed to engage Annie in a sensible conversation later that day, even though after a night of almost no sleep I was shattered myself. Annie was more forthcoming during this conversation as to how she had more frequently been feeling, both physically and mentally, and we were at least able to agree that she needed professional medical help.
Although I consider this after many years to have been the correct course of action to take, it has lead to numerous arguments and distressing periods in all of our lives.

How did I feel? As no diagnosis was immediately made, I was looking forward to seeing Annie, after a short period of hospital treatment, return to her old self and continue as a good wife and mother to our children. When the diagnosis was eventually given it is fair to say I was shell shocked. Severe mental illness didn't happen to people like us, with decent jobs, careers to look forward to, healthy children and a nice home. We weren't rich but were comfortable and had everything to look forward to. Why had this happened, was it the stress of work as Annie did work 3 nights a week

Annie Moon

as a nurse and we had two young children demanding as young kids are? We had a neighbour who we had had several rows with as they were your typical self righteous Christians and total hypocrites. They knew Annie worked nights but would constantly create unnecessary noise during the day depriving Annie of valuable sleep. Our oldest child was starting to become difficult with childminders and we were constantly having to find solutions to this. It has to be noted here that we received very little support from any close family- this has generally been a constant feature over all the many years of coming to terms with this illness. Were any one of these events or combinations to blame for Annie's illness? Who will ever know? It could have happened at anytime even without any of these turmoils in our lives. You can read all you like about mental illness and other than drugs or alcohol there is no obvious reasons as to who and why certain people are affected by it and others aren't.

I don't wish to go into detail on any of the situations I have had to deal with over the last 12 years or more, only that they have been distressing to all of us and, yes, I have to be truthful and admit there have been many times when I have been prepared to throw in the towel. Why didn't I? For many reasons which will not always be the same for other people out there; I loved Annie and had been very happy with her and hoped to recover this relationship fully. I have an old fashioned view of relationships/marriage; if

TO SCHIZOPHRENIA AND BACK

the person you have chosen to be your partner in life needs your help then it should be given until such time as it is made clear that it is not wanted in anyway anymore. We had 2 young children and I knew that it would be impossible for me alone to look after them, and there would be no help from family. I was concerned about how Annie would cope with them alone and what would happen if she had a relapse. There was no way I wanted my children to be taken into any sort of care even for short periods and I had an immediate distrust of Mental Health and Social Workers. I had to take the view that we could all beat this together and generally over the many years things have improved.

I would not want anyone reading this to think it has been nothing but a battle over the last 12 years as this is not the case. We have, in the main, managed to live a generally normal life, especially so over the last few years. Our children have grown up healthy and show no signs of having been overly affected by events; they are just your typical modern British teenagers and in many ways are better than other children we know who have had no traumatic events in their life. We have continued to live a comfortable life, still have our own house, car, have had many foreign holidays etc.
Annie is now in the final year of a degree course and will be returning to work within the next 12

Annie Moon

months. All this should help her deal with the illness. It has certainly been the case that whilst she as been studying her health and general outlook have improved massively as having something to concentrate on has prevented her from becoming bored and feeling worthless with no future to look forward to.

Most of my major gripes are more with the Medical profession and their approach to relatives of people affected by mental illness. They always have that convenient excuse of hiding behind the law and confidentially. This to me is a major issue that needs to be tackled as it is those closest to the sufferer that can first spot symptoms of relapse and take all the necessary steps to gain the correct help, but once the medical people get involved you are mostly pushed to the side and ignored. I have to admit that I have also often been very annoyed with Annie herself over the years for holding back many things from me, but I know the reasons and can half agree there was a case for them once but not now. It has taken me a long time to learn how to cope with some difficult and what can be demanding changes in behaviour and to still be able to continue with the normal other everyday stresses of modern life. There are still times when it does get too much for me but I have my own coping strategies; football, cycling, beers with the lads. We have both said many things over the years that we shouldn't have and we regret having done so but is this really any different from any other set of people?

TO SCHIZOPHRENIA AND BACK

Mental illness still carries a major stigma in society, yet is becoming increasingly common in varying degrees; the media do not help as any major incident of violence by a mentally ill person is always featured as a major issue. How many people though are killed or severely injured by a relative as against a mentally ill person? I grew up in the generation where people with problems were made fun of, and terms like "Schizo", "Loony", "Nutter" were said in jest but the world as moved on and people should be reassured that mentally ill people are not in the main dangerous and more likely to seek to be alone.

We still have our disputes and I still have to think is this the illness or just a typical domestic disagreement? But in the main the future is becoming increasingly brighter and I hope that it can continue in this way.

One member of my family, Ruth, has been a good support over the years. On many occasions we would walk Simba over the moors and along the canals. We would drink coffee and chat. It was Ruth who recommended that I keep a diary whilst I wasn't feeling myself. It was this diary that I showed to the doctors involved in my treatment

Annie Moon

and ultimately it played a part in my diagnosis.

TO SCHIZOPHRENIA AND BACK

CHAPTER 5

PSYCHOSIS

Exerts from my diary
No 1 and No 2 are my children; I have not put their names down to protect their identity.

**GOD
BLESS
YOU**

**ANNIE
MARY-JANE
MOON**

Miss prim and proper

Thursday 16th February 1995 1600hrs

Just got up after a night shift.

I am not stupid, although people like to judge me before they know me. I know that they talk about me and laugh or make 'snidey' comments. I have to keep my mouth shut lately as stupid things may come out: the snake and the Lord is my shepherd

Annie Moon

I shall not want he maketh me lie down in green pastures and leadeth me to the moors to lie down in the rain and be levitated up to God.

I know that I am not thinking straight but I can't suppress it forever as it gives me terrible headaches and then the rats come, I know that they are not real, but they're there and its doing my f****** head in. It used to start in the car when the radio was on, the 'Pogues' and the 'Who' willed me to the reservoirs, I'd be alright after sitting up there for a few hours in the car.

Book, I want to sleep but I wake up with headaches, I know that my brain is being taken away from me, bit by bit from the hole by the side of my head.

I am frightened of speaking out- they'd love it wouldn't they- they always said she was a mental case.

I know that if I go to the moors to see God, they'll come for me- I can't speak out because the children are so well balanced, I don't want to frighten them.

Miss neurotics at it again **this book will burst into flames once out of my possession** and they **won't** be able to get at **her** mind.

I can't go to work now without seeing the spiders on the ceilings and the walls, all the patients have

TO SCHIZOPHRENIA AND BACK

something to say about her.

Mary, Mary quite contrary how does your garden grow?

I am sure there is a dead baby under the concrete floor at my house, sometimes the smell is bad. The council say that it must be the drains.

Write, write, write away, never time to rest or play.

SHUSH, SHUSH, SHUSH

I've seen the spaceship over the moors

A can of pop, dibbley dop.

I can't function properly.

My husband is wonderful, I love him so much but I can't tell him about my thoughts, it will drive him away- he'll compare **her**, with the natural mother.

I feel so much better writing this, my headache is lifting, it's got to come out!!!!!!!!!

I love my children and I would never harm them, my bug gun is damaged now, so I have no defences for them and now No 1's poorly.

Bye Bye

Annie Moon

X Annie

Thursday 16th February 1995 1800hrs

Just started tea, my heads throbbing again and my mind is racing- be normal, be normal, smile-

I keep feeling the need to lie on the moors- it's raining heavily- it's so helpful to write this down- I feel that I am not alone. I can talk to you book and you will not judge, condemn me or liquefy my brains! You cannot **LABEL** me.

Huh, somebody asked if I took drugs yesterday- **how insulting!** I felt really hurt, (really hurt), I feel quite low now.

Go to jail do not pass go

FLOWERS   FLOWERS   FLOWERS   FLOWERS
FLOWERS   FLOWERS   FLOWERS   FLOWERS
FLOWERS   FLOWERS   FLOWERS
FLOWERS
                    FLOWERS   FLOWERS
                        FLOWERS

Who do I trust?

My husband with my life *providing he has a tattoo and a birthmark*

Mark

TO SCHIZOPHRENIA AND BACK

M*

D*****

Nobody else can know me I will not allow it.

All others are liars, two faced, hypocrites out for themselves.

10pm Thursday

My heads banging again, Todd's quiet again, I know he's cross with me, I want to relax with him but my head is XXXX
$$\begin{array}{c}XXXX\\XXXX\end{array}$$
Goodnight God Bless

PS Supposed to be in work tonight, but I know I'll start being stupid. (I imagined myself in a long grey dress in the 18th century last night).

Friday 17th February 1995 0730hrs

I have just got up, I slept from 11pm until 2am and woke up with a 'funny' head. I slept until 3am and then No2 woke me up so I went into his bed. This morning my headache is only slight and I feel very embarrassed at what I have written although she is still trying to make my brain 'funny'. I will not let

Annie Moon

her get the better of me this morning.

Todd said that married couples are supposed to sleep in the same bed to No2. It's a bit difficult for me when he's climbing on my head in the night.

Friday 0805hrs

She's starting again- I wish she'd go away! I've got to get my head straight and sort the boys out.

('She' being an auditory and visual hallucination, also referred to as MJ).
I went to see our family doctor the other day to help No1, I asked for a sick note but he wanted to know why- its not normal for a doctor to take his pet snake in when he's seeing children- it didn't bother the boys though.

Mother rang last night. **I will not answer the phone now I can't stand it!** You never know who's listening in, anyway people only want to gossip or talk about themselves. Todd can fob them off.

THE WICKED WITCH IS DEAD

I feel <u>sad</u> now

Not a tear shall be shed

TO SCHIZOPHRENIA AND BACK

For the thoughts in my head

Go away
Go away
Go away

<u>Friday 1100hrs</u>

Back from town, it says in the paper that God will meet me on Wednesday but I have to be careful until then. I feel ready now- we will go together book, I will transfer all my money to Toddy so that he does not get taxed on it.

I can feel the grass and the night air already, I love to see the lights.

My cold sore is going now, so they can't get into the house to put their needle into my head anymore.

Bang   Bang   Bang

<u>Friday 1330hrs</u>

Some cheeky bast*** has sent me a leaflet about a listening service- how dare they!!!! They are taking the pi**, what can they expect when some of your brain is liquid? I wish I knew who it was- I have my suspicions. My head is aching, I don't know if I can wait till Wednesday.

(I felt very angry when I wrote this).

Saturday 18th February 1995 0010hrs

Dear book, I feel a lot better, I've just come down from the moors, 5 hours I waited- he didn't come- I have no headache, I feel quite depressed-I just want to drive around xxx

I'll wait a bit longer…

Saturday 0400hrs

Book, I'm a lot warmer now. I've decided that if it takes too much longer for him to come I'm going to have to go up the pylon.

Saturday 0400hrs (cont)

Off weeee go …3 circuits of the county.

Saturday 1520hrs

The tree was very nice and the wires tried their best, but there was not enough rain.

TO SCHIZOPHRENIA AND BACK

We will see how it is on Wednesday

Todd said that he saw my step mum and dad, I felt very intruded and agitated- I don't want to know, they are **not** part of me.

Todd asked me if I love him, of course I do, but it takes too much effort to talk.

Sunday 19th February 1995 12noon

Dear book, they must have come in the night and hurt my ankle, to stop me going on Wednesday- they're evil, they'll try to kill me if they can

MJ said it would be alright without my cold sore.

I can feel the electricity running through my body- I'm scared.

My head is hurting.

MJ tried to get me to jump into the reservoir.

Sunday 8.05pm

I have my defences ready, they <u>will not</u> experiment on me!!!

Annie Moon

It's so hard waiting.

Monday 20th February 12.30pm

I felt 'back to normal' from 7pm till bedtime last night, Mary Jane (MJ), didn't try to bother me.

I closed my eyes at midnight and I woke every hour on the hour.

No1 son asked if we could all go swimming together this week. I may not be here.

MJ wanted to push Toddy's head under the water- she can't touch you book.

I have more free will than <u>that.</u>

Monday 1815hrs

I have seen Family doctor- I feel as though I have signed my own death warrant.

Mary Jane, I'm so sorry to have betrayed you. I will sort it out.

Xxxxxxxxxxxxxxxxxxxxxxxxxxxxxxxxxxxxxxxxxxxxxx
xxxxxxxxxxxxxxxxxxxxxxxxxxxxxxxxxxxxxxxxxxxxxx
xxxxxxxxxxxxxxxxxxxxxxxxxxxxxxxxxxxxxxxxxxxxxx
xxxxx

TO SCHIZOPHRENIA AND BACK

Tuesday 21st February 1710hrs

I am absolutely furious and I feel that I could scream and shout and I do not know why.

I feel vexed, violent and abhorrent.

Tuesday 2300hrs

I know why- I've just come back from dropping No1 son off at a party in town and everyone was looking at me and saying terrible things about me because I was ignoring No2 sons screams (out of temper and tiredness).

Toddy keeps going on about doctors, I really don't want to see a psychiatrist- I don't feel that I need to- I wish that he'd never seen you book, but he did go in my bag without asking.

I am sorry that I distressed Toddy earlier but my body just shook with anger. He said that he'd spoken to my step mum- I felt agitated again. I asked him never to mention her name

Annie Moon

He understands that I like to unplug the phone so that bad things can't come down the wire and into my house.

I may ask him tomorrow if he would like to come up to the moors, to see God, he'll understand then.

Just these last few days, I have 'jumped out of my skin' when Toddy or the boys have come up to me.

Family doctor asked me the other day if-huh it was yesterday! (I've lost track of time and reality)- if I had thought about suicide. A few weeks ago I wanted to die- for absolutely no reason at all. I have a lovely house, wonderful husband and children and a well paid job.

I know however that I cannot commit suicide, as a suicidal soul is forever in turmoil; one must go naturally i.e. of expenditure on the moors, then God can either take you or leave you depending on whether he's ready for you or not.

Tuesday 2300hrs (cont)

MJ's behaved very well tonight- not a murmur since 8pm.

TO SCHIZOPHRENIA AND BACK

I'm glad that R*** is there for Toddy and the boys, she's quite human.

Wednesday 22nd February 1995 @1100hrs

I am at Animal Zone. I couldn't stand being in the queue and got quite agitated. I spoke sharply to the boys.

It is extremely crowded, so I have found a quiet spot and I am sitting on the floor. I have my headphones on; I do not feel that I am here- I feel like an outsider looking in. My mind is never still.

She gets so agitated with other people – F*** OFF, F*** OFF she is saying

I have seen a few 'friends', I have done my best to avoid them, I don't want to talk. Conversation is so false; people say one thing and think another.

I feel very philosophical and like a spirit visiting the earth- maybe I am, maybe I'm not meant to be here for too long.

Number 1 is such a good boy, he has looked after Number 2 for me; I have told him how I feel about his good behaviour here and he will be rewarded.

I love you book.

Annie Moon

Next door said that our house was plagued by bad luck, maybe the baby under the concrete is not at rest, I have heard it crying in the past- they think that it's a figure of speech that I am using- if I could I would have the foundations ripped out by the police, its too easy for people to get away with things like that.

Annie Moon

It's good to see the boys having so much fun.

Wednesday 2000hrs

Consultant Psychiatrist 1 has been tonight, my fear and apprehensions of freedom removed, straight jackets, electrocution, drug stupors have all been dispelled- he didn't <u>appear</u> to judge me. The moors seem a long way away tonight.

MJ you are to die, at The hospital no 1!

I feel that I am sponging off the benefactors of any treatment- which I still <u>don't</u> really want or need!

My headache is quite bad tonight.

I am frightened of being poisoned.

TO SCHIZOPHRENIA AND BACK

Wednesday 2130hrs

Good night god bless you book.

Wednesday 2255hrs

I've just woken up- she says they're going to poison me- I don't want to go- the electricity is running through my body again…they're going to poison you!!!!!!!!

She awoke me again in the night but I can't remember why.

Thursday 23rd February I went into a private hospital

(I went into a private hospital because I worked for the National Health Service; our hospital had an arrangement for them to look after the hospital staff privately).

Thursday 2200hrs

I have just calmed down, I have been bombarded by questions and all I want is to be left alone and

Annie Moon

to go home.

I feel as though they are laughing at me.

Why? Just because I want to sit in the dark did one nurse laugh... it really upset me.

The orange juice has a white powder floating on top of it.

I want to go home

My head is aching.

I must say the room is lovely.

(The following was written in very distorted handwriting at the time due to the antipsychotic medication that they had given me at the hospital).

Friday 0130hrs

I feel settled now; I've had a pill- I can't believe that I've not got a headache!

Friday PM

Saw Consultant Psychiatrist no 2.

I felt very agitated pm, very angry and violent. I

TO SCHIZOPHRENIA AND BACK

don't know why, I went for a walk to try and get rid of it but I thought I saw a woman in the tree waving at me to remind me that she's still there.

Since I've been taking the tablets she's not bothered me, although I feel she is still trying to get into my mind- I wish she'd go away.

I have not stopped sleeping, it is **utter bliss!!!**

Sunday 26th February 1995

She's not been today.

Sunday 1330hrs

She came to the dining room window, I feel very agitated and upset- the nurse gave me a tablet and I felt ok.

Todd and the boys came for tea.

Monday 1330 February 27th 1995

Felt overwhelmingly sad for no real reason at all.

I kept saying to myself PULL YOURSELF TOGETHER!!

Annie Moon

She's tried to come but I won't encourage her.

1645hrs

Can't concentrate to write up essay (I was in the middle of a nursing course and had some work to finish off).

I've seen her in the field, she is angry. I feel that she wants to take me away.

I feel distraught- really I don't know why.

It helps book, to write it all down.
(my handwriting was very poor due to the drugs).

Monday 2045hrs

Feel a lot better after talking to A, my key worker. I felt sure that I would be better off at home but she is so kind and reassuring she put my abstract thoughts into perspective.

NOT HAD A HEADACHE FOR 3 DAYS

Tuesday 2045hrs

I've felt ok today- for some unknown reason felt

TO SCHIZOPHRENIA AND BACK

overwhelmed with emotion during occupational health- A gave me some chlorpromazine- I felt so fine after this that I managed to write up some of my essay.

I still think however that I would be better off on the moors rather than taking tablets.
No headache today

PS I still can't watch television properly.

Wednesday 1st March 1995 0500hrs

Awoke twice, had a cup of tea both times- <u>I felt fine, very, very fine!</u> I awoke without <u>her</u> help.

MJ has gone- I feel very sad at losing her, I also feel quite resentful at the Dr and nurses for killing her even though I know that <u>she was all</u> the badness in me.

Wednesday 2030hrs

I felt really good all afternoon, but, I've had a couple of hours sleep and I feel very restless and agitated and wanting to go home again.

My headache has started again.

Annie Moon

Thursday 2nd March 1995 0005hrs

This is the time it happened. I could smell cigarette smoke on my pyjamas, my bedding and in my hair- I thought that it must be coming from the day room via the pipes the plugs and the cracks in the door, I sprayed deodorant around and opened the windows- nurse gave me another sleeping tablet and some painkillers for my headache

I slept till 6am.

Felt great this am.

Thursday 1145hrs

I feel very agitated- I don't want them poisoning me with pills- I want to go home!!!!!!
Thursday 1300hrs

They wouldn't let me go home; they think that I am mad. Consultant Psychiatrist no 2 thinks I am, he's sectioned me for 3 days, to get another doctor's advice before I go home.

Friday 3rd March 1995 0845hrs

I feel as fit as a fiddle, although I am very restless!

TO SCHIZOPHRENIA AND BACK

Friday 1130hrs

I feel ok, a bit low and wanting to go home. I want life to be as it was.

I have been to exercise class and weekend planning.

Friday 1820hrs? 3rd March

My general practitioner Family doctor and a social worker interviewed me. I have to stay for treatment.

I have no feelings- I feel numb tonight.

Another doctor came, I have been detained on a section 2 of the Mental Health Act for 28 days

(From what I can remember I told them about MJ in the reservoir beckoning me to join her and me wanting to wander the moors).

Some of my friends came and made me laugh.

Saturday 4th March 1995 1330hrs

Annie Moon

Slept really well- didn't have medication except for 20mg Temazepam because my mouth and eyes are dry.

I felt low this morning but feel really good now. I feel ok to go home.

Saturday 1400hrs

Absolutely gutted, B** my new room mate asked me if I was a spy because I was writing in my book.

(I was crying inconsolably at the dining room table).

Saturday 2030hrs

Feeling better now, lying in bed. I feel 'normal' and believe it or not I have managed to watch a whole program on T.V, although I don't want to talk to anybody if I can help it.

It seems that my mood is

HIGH   ----------------------------

NORMAL---

TO SCHIZOPHRENIA AND BACK

LOW

       0600hrs   0900hrs
12-1500hrs   BEDTIME

Sunday 5th March 1995 0800hrs

Awoke at 0600hrs, thinking that somebody was trying to wake me up by coughing, i.e. hm, cough, hm. M the nurse said that another nurse had just been in checking on everybody.

I managed another half an hour of sleep then I awoke thinking that there was a big piece of root ginger on the floor with insects in it. I asked M for my tablets early when I got the courage to come out of my room. I lay on the bed and had 'ideas' that there was a huge fly had its eyes next to mine. That feeling has gone now- I feel ok.

Sunday 5th March 1730hrs

I am very upset. I feel as though I want MJ back so that I can go into the reservoir with her. Toddy has been, with the boys – he is saying that I can have 2 moor weeks then he'll appeal. The boys fight and scream and the doctors say that I must stay in for 4 weeks.

Annie Moon

I want to be on my own.

I want to be left alone.

Monday 6th March

I feel wonderful but shaky

Monday 1800hrs

No mood swings. Blood pressure 80/60, feel ok, but head aches when sitting and standing and I feel faint all the time.

Tuesday 7th March 1995 0900hrs

(Some of the entries in this diary had questionable dates, as I had forgotten which month it was and which day of the week. I have corrected these days to ensure the accuracy and continuity).

I feel like they're trying to kill me. These tablets make me so dizzy, I feel as though my heart will stop and I will die, but they're not listening to me- I have been brought here to die.

I feel despondent.

TO SCHIZOPHRENIA AND BACK

Tuesday 0950hrs

I feel very agitated, I don't know why. I feel that I can't sit still. Last night I felt like walking to the moors. My head aches.

Tuesday 1120hrs

Still very agitated- I want to pace up and down, but my head feels like 'cotton wool'. I want to go home <u>RIGHT NOW!</u> Every time I walk I feel faint. I've found it very difficult just to make a cup of tea.

I feel as though I am drunk.

Seen Consultant Psychiatrist no 2. I feel happier now that he has changed my medication.

Tuesday 1800hrs

Saw a man slumped on some garden debris- I thought am I seeing things or is he hurt. The staff nurse said that it was plastic. I felt oh no, I'm losing my mind! I feel very despondent. I want to see God on the moors.

Tuesday night

I got very upset when the boys went home.

I stayed up late. I had the start of some 'thoughts', so I asked for my medication and they went, my head was clear.

Wednesday 8th March 1995 0500hrs

Awoke to a bad dream, had a cup of tea.

Wednesday 0730hrs

Woke up feeling wonderful- no dizziness, they have changed my tablets.

Wednesday 1600hrs

In pottery and feeling agitated, I don't know why- calm yourself Annie or else you'll never get home!!!!

I want to go home and to the moors.

TO SCHIZOPHRENIA AND BACK

RIGHT ENOUGH IS ENOUGH!

PSYCHO ANALYSING TIME

A, my key worker had to calm me down this evening because I wanted to go home to my children.

1) **AM I DEPRESSED?**
2) **WHO IS MJ?**
3) **WHAT ARE THE THINGS I SEE?**
4) **MY THOUGHTS**
5) **MY FUTURE**
6) **THE MOORS**

1. AM I DEPRESSED?

No, maybe I was but now I'm not, I am taking charge of my life, behaving like responsible adult, parent and worker. I pine for my children which is only natural.

2. WHO IS MJ?

MJ is obviously a part of my mind- women just don't appear in trees!

I think that she was a response to my personal

distress, at being overworked and overtired. She was an outlet for all my negative thoughts, as I, as a person, do not swear, do not believe in suicide, do not focus physical anger on people, things- I made 'MJ' to do this for me and while she was there she was to some extent a comfort for me.

3. THE THINGS I SEE.

I admit to myself that I saw things that weren't there.

I don't know why these things happened- but when they did, I usually had a terrible headache.

The man slumped over debris was a misinterpretation of what I could see due to uncertainty about my senses because of my previous state of mind and also my failing eyesight.

4. MY THOUGHTS.

The telephone- when people ring, they usually use me as an agony aunt for all their woes. If not woes then for gossip, slander etc.

I just wanted a rest from this and during my distorted thoughts time I described this as 'badness' coming down the telephone line.

I know the anatomy of a plug and plug sockets and I know that smoke can't come out of them- my

TO SCHIZOPHRENIA AND BACK

mind was greatly distressed.

5. MY FUTURE.

I want to go home, be a mother, wife and nurse.

We are to go on holiday abroad when I go home.

I have no desire to die.

I would like to spend more time with my children, by changing the amount of hours I do at work.

I love life, I love spring, summer, autumn and winter- the only thing that makes me miserable is drizzling rain.

6. THE MOORS

The moors for me is tranquillity, peace and quiet.

I know that God cannot come through the high tension cables, but I thought that when I was distressed.

I swear to God, If Consultant Psychiatrist no 2 lets me home I will follow his medication instructions as I know it has helped to rest my mind and stop my, I suppose 'delusions'.

I wouldn't like to repeat this episode in my life, it has been very scary.

Thursday 9th March 2100hrs

I've felt wonderful/fine all day!

I feel that the contents of this book are someone else's thoughts. *(I am referring to the diary)*

Friday 10th March 1995 1900hrs

I have felt fine all day.

I have seen Consultant Psychiatrist no 2. He says that I can go home for a short spell over the weekend- yipeeeeeeee!!!!!!!!!!!!

Saturday 11th March

Slept very well with 20mg Temazepam. Went home for the day- <u>lovely</u>! Only thoughts were to snap out of my tiredness, probably due to the Haloperidol 5mg. Thought I saw A in my home town- nonsense. I walked for ½ an hour this morning. Felt as though the police were in

TO SCHIZOPHRENIA AND BACK

unmarked cars on the motorway watching me.

Sunday 12th March 1995 2215

I slept for most of the day- muscles restless, so I had a tablet to stop the shakes. I was not hungry today. I feel low in mood tonight for no particular reason- I just want to put my headphones on and be alone.

Painted a picture after my anti- shake tablet- watched a <u>full</u> TV film!! My concentration is back.

I want to be outside alone; the moors don't come into it. I want my music.

I want to ring mum- but I know I can't, she'll only hurt me in times to come.

It's been a while since I have wanted my music on, I feel that MJ is coming back, but I mustn't let anyone know or I'll never get home from hospital.

Monday 13th March

I feel much better this morning. I had about 4 hours sleep, I woke up to a bad dream at 5am. Today I want to post a letter, buy some herbal tea bags and something else, (I've forgotten what) at

Annie Moon

the village. Oh yes a face pack.

That badness was in my head last night; I feel that my sleep has made me a stronger person to deal with it.

I went to the community meeting (*group therapy*) at 2.30pm, I couldn't stand it, I couldn't concentrate, I feel like an outsider who has no business or need for stress management.

Some of the residents are really poorly. I am not one of them.

Head phones time. I am not sad just very agitated….the bear went over the mountain, to see what he could see.

I want to go home and to the moors; I feel really peeved.

It's such a lovely day I could get lost on the moors.

God will be with me up there. He cannot reach me here; there are too many people to get through I can always hear children outside the hospital windows playing ring 'o' ring 'o' roses.

TO SCHIZOPHRENIA AND BACK

**LOVE THY
NEIGHBOUR**

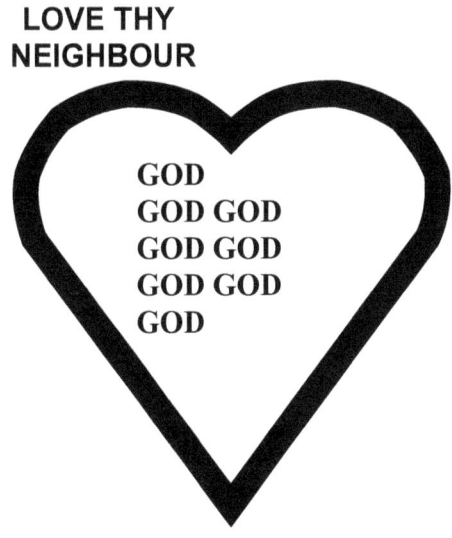

OK OK OK OK OK OK OK OK OK OK OK OK OK OK OK OK OK OK OK

I'm sat here with my head phones; it's nice to be amongst people as a spectator not being included in communication.

(At different stages in my diary I would write my signature as if I was signing an official document).

Tuesday 14th March

I had a good nights sleep, I only awoke a few times, I took a sleeping tablet at midnight.

Annie Moon

I have a headache this morning and I saw the medical officer because I couldn't pass urine (*this was due to some medication that I was taking*), I am also constipated. I managed to pee 150mls, I am writing it like this because I am now on a chart.

My mood is good, except for my headache.

I love life.

Is MJ a spirit? I think so!

Tuesday 14<u>th</u> 1230hrs

I feel very positive. Could it be that somebody has used black magic on me in revenge?

I really thought that I had a baby, dead or alive in my womb

Tuesday pm

Felt really good in the evening. I ran about outside and in the games room with the boys.

I do appreciate ad love my husband x.

TO SCHIZOPHRENIA AND BACK

Wednesday 15th March 1995 1545hrs

Slept for a total of 7 hours on and off- kept waking up due to coughing.

Felt fine all day.

I have been to all of the programmed classes, I have played table tennis with another patient/resident/client and I have just walked to the village and back- just under an hours walk. No odd feelings!

I felt agitated @ 8pm- had a fight with a male resident.

I was very upset because it brought back feelings from when I was younger.

Thursday 16th March 1800hrs

I felt very, very tired all day. I even woke up with a headache after having 20mg Temazepam last night.

I saw MJ for a matter of seconds prior to lunch-there were no children and she was crying. I asked for a Chlorpromazine (*antipsychotic*), - these make my eyes sticky. I prefer the haloperidol. Felt ok after, still slurring my words and forgetting things etc.

Friday17th March 1995

Slept, slept, slept!!!! No thoughts

Saturday18th March 1995

Brill!! Went home, went to the shops and the library. The boys had their hair cut at the barbers. We went to the park and to visit my Dad and step mum. I had a mobile hairdresser come and cut my hair… it's very nice to be home. I have been very well looked after. I even went for a ½ hour walk and picked some daffodils.

Sunday 19th March

Muscles were twitching in my buttocks so I took some Procyclidine, the tablets helped slightly.

Went to Dads for a meal, how could I think my step mum was against me, she is so kind and considerate.

TO SCHIZOPHRENIA AND BACK

Feeling well all weekend. I <u>even</u> took my tablets. No upsetting thoughts, no desire to go up to the moors- my mind is normal. I have no ambition now to get my degree in 18 months- it can be spread out, I'll still be here.

I am not going to rush at anything, like I have been doing.

I even checked Consultant Psychiatrist no 2's history in the library, I feel so privileged to be under his care.

Monday 20th March

Slept well, no medication needed, went to exercises, walked to the village, went running.

Felt quite 'manic' today.

I feel ready for home.

Tuesday 21st March

No thoughts- feeling very homesick, very bored, restless and tired.

Friday 24th March 1995

Annie Moon

Came home yesterday for weekend leave. I've cut the tablets down because of this restless feeling that I keep getting. As a result of my reduction in medication and my restlessness I have started with diarrhoea, I also feel very 'panicky'.

Saturday 25<u>th</u>

Cut the tablets right down, I felt suicidal because I didn't want to put my family through years of torment... I rang the hospital up for support and they were very helpful.

Sunday 26<u>th</u> (Mothers day)

Poor nights sleep- head starting again-'buzzing', had a lovely day, did some housework etc.

27<u>th</u> March 1995

No tablets, felt as though my head was 'hollow'. I went for a swim and a sauna with my step mum. I drove the car, felt great after a couple of 'odd' hours.

Tuesday 28<u>th</u> March

It snowed heavily today. I went back to the

TO SCHIZOPHRENIA AND BACK

hospital. I felt trapped again, persecuted and doomed.

I spoke to Consultant Psychiatrist no 2 again today with regards to my medication's side effects. He changed them to Thioridizine 25mg four times a day.

I packed my suitcase and went to bed fully clothed; I thought that if I did that then they could not stop me from going home.

Wednesday 27th March

Felt weepy, paranoid and dizzy this morning even though I slept well last night.

Spoke to my birth mother and she feels that we all go 'funny' at 26- 27years of age. Nobby with drugs, my younger brother with his law breaking and immoral behaviour and my elder sister, according to my birth mother, saw God himself when she gave birth to one of her children.

She said that we all go at 100 miles per hour, it's in our genes.

Please god I hope that my children are ok.

Huh, put my t-shirt on back to front this morning.

COMING TO TERMS

Sunday 18th June, (Fathers day) 1995

Sulpiride 200mg BD

I looked up the tablets that I am on a few weeks ago in the drugs book and what they are for, they are for schizophrenia. I asked my general practitioner Family doctor if that's what I have been 'burdened' with. He said that it was schizophrenia. I resigned myself to this and got some books out of the library and even though I

TO SCHIZOPHRENIA AND BACK

couldn't read them- the words are too much for me to take in- I managed to pick up on the headlines etc and noticed that diet was an important factor- mainly gluten free- so I'll give that a go I thought. Then 3 days ago I thought I don't have schizophrenia, I'm just maladjusted, so I stopped the tablets. I was feeling very tired, as well, even though I have done very well sleeping this last week.

I am writing this to remind me how I feel into my 3rd day without medication. I feel weepy- for absolutely no reason- I have said time and time again that I go 'funny' when I am listening to music, as if the sound waves affect my brain somehow, but people just think I'm 'potty'.

I want to lie on the moors, but I keep thinking of Toddy and the boys. It is so easy to lose everything you've worked towards. I also keep thinking that I am pregnant. I know I can't be, maybe its some kind of subconscious desire to have more children- I would love a little girl, but Toddy doesn't want any more and besides which it would be quite irresponsible to bring more children into the world with a mother who has a history of mental illness- they could inherit it. It just wouldn't be fair on them.

I'm even producing milk, I think that maybe it's the medication. I have a very slight brown discharge,

Annie Moon

down below. I'm thinking maybe I've lost a twin or have a chocolate cyst- the sensible half of me says don't be silly, you're 2 weeks into your menstrual cycle and these things happen when you ovulate.

I also keep thinking maybe I'm not able to concentrate properly because I breast fed my children for a total of 4 years, and did after all only stop feeding No2 son last summer after 2 1/2 years- obscene I know, but the trials and tribulations of depriving a youngster of his comforter were just too much.

Anyway 1 1/2 hours after taking my tablet, I feel OK-

- a note to remind me I do not always think like this. I am quite a normal, happy go lucky person when my head is not full of rubbish and I do not always dwell on myself- I've got too much to do and 2 lovely boys and a good husband to live for- not that suicide is an option.

I've even started to keep fit! Even though it's <u>killing</u> me.

I hate what I have written it is so **pathetic!!!!!**

July 4th 1995

I have a headache. I am distraught today for no

TO SCHIZOPHRENIA AND BACK

reason and crying to music **PATHETIC.**

I just want to put my head phones on and shut myself away from everybody; it's only been 2 days without medication. I feel that I can't look after anyone else. I can't stand it when people want to talk to me.

<u>It's not getting any better.</u>

I can't face the chores that I have to do. When I am on the tablets they are not a problem, yet with the tablets, I have had a non stop period for 1 month and I've put on weight.

I feel overcrowded at home. Toddy can't sleep lately, he is waking early- he needs a good rest.

I've got to keep on this line: -
=======================================

I can't make conversation; it's too much hard work and quite meaningless.

<u>2100hrs</u>

I've had 2 tablets, I don't feel uptight now. How long is it going to take before I can do a million things at one time again?

Annie Moon

I just feel emotionless.

Friday 21st July 1995

I can't remember when I last took my drugs, but I have felt fine for a few days/? Weeks, until Toddy upset me last night. We had a wonderful time at A*'s birthday party and then for no reason, Toddy went into 'cut off mode', as if it was wrong for me to enjoy myself. I cannot cope with hostility from someone whom I love, when I try to please them and not me- this went on until sleep.

In the morning he wanted a kiss goodbye, as if it is alright to switch on and off. This made me very upset and fed up with trying to please- why should I! People only treat you like dirt.

I was OK this morning when Mark came round to visit. Around dinner time I couldn't stop sobbing and wanting to seriously die, taking the children with me to save them from the hurt they will get just by living- people can be so nasty. Mad M**** was always nice one minute and wicked the next.

(*I was very low at this point and have never at any other time in my life right up until now 2004 ever wanted to harm my children*).
It's so hurtful when you try so hard to please.

I thought, you're not psychotic, you're depressed, I

TO SCHIZOPHRENIA AND BACK

only took a *!* (*tablet*) when I thought that the house was cursed.

I felt I needed to talk to somebody, a doctor maybe, but I knew they would say 'take your pills' and the children would go on the 'At Risk Register'.

I bided my time to see if I would feel differently after a while- I went to My CPN's and an hour after taking the *!* (*tablet*) I felt fine only so upset that I thought of ending it all, only a matter of hours ago I was thinking of drugging us all and I would go somewhere quiet and use carbon monoxide gas, it would have only taken minutes, the boys would be free from a life of misery and conceit and Toddy could start a new life.

(My children are my life, I can only say I had hit rock bottom, I felt that life was bad and that there was a better deal going on in heaven, later in the years to come I would often feel that it would be better for everyone if I was dead but I have never ever thought about harming my children since).

What now? I am not depressed, Toddy apologised for his behaviour and told me how much he loved me and how he stood by me whilst I was in hospital- I spent most of my time worrying about him and the boys- I AM A VERY GRATEFUL PERSON!!!!!!!!

Annie Moon

I feel fine now as if my feelings come in waves and a switch is being turned on and off.

I love my family- Toddy, No1 and No2.

P.S I won the skipping race yesterday in the mum's event at sports day at the boy's school.

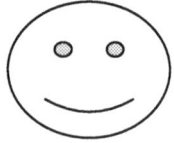

I FEEL BRILLIANT

Saturday 2nd December 1995 4.30pm

Last week, whilst taking my medication as prescribed, i.e. Sulpiride 200mg in the morning and 400mg at night, I started to smell the baby rotting, I smelled smoke and allsorts- it concerned me greatly. CPN has still not been in touch after being referred 8 weeks ago.

TO SCHIZOPHRENIA AND BACK

Today I have been off the tablets for 8 days- I have felt great all week, this is the first time in a while that I have wanted to take off to the moors, it has lasted 2 hours and has now passed- I felt weepy for no reason. I haven't done that for a while and now I feel fine again. I feel fresh and have done all week. I am keeping on top of my housework and cleaning for my step mum. I have an appointment on 11th December with occupational health with regards to work. I feel animosity towards Consultant Psychiatrist 1 after what he has written about me and I just hope that I can control myself when I go to the ECT suite, where occupational health is. I also keep thinking that my birth mother is going to get in touch, she is evil and wicked and tells lies- I hope that she stays away.

I want to go wandering. Denial of schizophrenia is the best way of coping at the moment; maybe I have to go through some sort of grieving process.

Sunday 3rd December 1995

I feel that my mind is stuck and I can't get on with things because I'm thinking too much, especially about not taking my tablets. What will happen if I let things get worse- I will lose my family and my home- so I am going to take one and see how I feel- I wish that they made Sulpiride in injections.

Annie Moon

Having just swallowed the tablet, I feel happy already, I know that this must be psychological, it's as if I'm testing myself to see if I am cured, last week I thought I was; before it took only 2 days to become weepy and paranoid etc, now it has taken 8 days- surely this is a good sign.

P.S. sleeping well, probably due to my night caps! (2 glasses of home made wine)- only while I'm off my tablets.

I will write a book about this one day.

P.S. I can't stand Todd's wanting to be alone 'cut off mode', when I'm not on my tablets I feel that I need constant reassurance of his love- I know he likes to be quiet when the boys have hassled him or he's tired but I always think that he has fallen out with me because of something that I have done- I feel stressed then and I want to go somewhere alone- to the moors. *(This was to be nearer to God, I was very paranoid at these times. I felt that he could communicate with me through the power cables).*

Monday 4th December 1995

Feeling very suicidal- I feel as if I've failed. I worry for my children's future.

TO SCHIZOPHRENIA AND BACK

Tuesday 5th December 1995

Felt ok this morning- I felt weepy when I spoke to a Community Psychiatric nurse over the phone. I've started taking the Prozac again. Feeling alright in the afternoon.

Wednesday 5th - Monday 11th December 1995

Felt fine all week, however, I hardly moved off the couch on Saturday- I can't get my head awake.

Monday 11th December 1995

I saw the occupational health doctor, he said that I could go back to work, although I must work fewer hours and no nights. I was very pleased but worried about financial implications and childcare arrangements.

Tuesday 12th December 1995

I want to retire on ill health grounds; the thought of going back to work and mixing with people is keeping me awake and giving me diarrhoea.

Annie Moon

Thursday 14th December 1995

Saw Family doctor my general practitioner about retiring, he says no.

Friday 15th December 1995

Couldn't move off the couch again today, I couldn't get my head awake- it's quite distressing for me; how am I going to stay awake at work.

Saturday16th-Wednesday 20th December 1995

Started wanting to stop pills again- still nervous.

January 2nd 1996

Started feeling pills are causing my blood to turn to powder in my legs. Consultant Psychiatrist 1 is a liar and is not a doctor and he knows that I know because I've been to the library. He's just a black belt at Karate and I am not afraid, I will punch his face in- he thinks that holding his plastic roof over his head means something. He's been against me all the way and doesn't want me nursing. *(Consultant Psychiatrist 1, is a lovely man, I was*

TO SCHIZOPHRENIA AND BACK

not myself when I wrote this).

I went to work today. A Polish man said that I only gave him whisky because I'd done f*** all all day and that I was trying to get them all drunk so that they wouldn't notice! He was smiling sweetly when he said it. *(I believe now that I was having auditory hallucinations and that he wouldn't have said those things).*

I felt anger towards the pharmacists because they didn't answer the bell quickly enough and the room was full of people looking. I wanted to shout 'get a f***ing move on you b***ards but I was just off hand with them, I managed not to make a scene.

I FEEL THAT EVERYONE KNOWS WHAT I AM THINKING!!!!!!

I am worried that if I tell of my thoughts they will keep me away from my boys.

I don't want to go and see Consultant Psychiatrist 1 at the end of January, I know that I won't be able to control myself. I just want to punch his face in and where will that get me- no job-a criminal record- children upset- plus he'd say that his diagnosis was correct-that would just prove him right. I want to stay away, but occupational health say that I must see him- I feel very stressed about

Annie Moon

this.

I feel worried about going to see CPN's on Monday, I feel that if I go I won't be able to see my boys on No2's birthday.

I just want to go to work and stay away from psychiatric people.

Wednesday 3rd of January 1996

Felt buzzing this am- can't remember what I was thinking but I know that it wasn't right. I feel as though I should try the monthly injection, but I'm scared of it- but I feel as though......- I can't remember what I was going to write!

2200hrs feel 'normal', I will see how I go on.
EXASPERATED!!!!!!!!!!!!!!!!!!

6 MONTHS LATER
Wednesday 31st July 1996

(First day of injection; this injection is supposed to take over from having to take tablets orally. Its effects last longer; for some people up to a month). Felt fine; also had chlorpromazine this am.

TO SCHIZOPHRENIA AND BACK

Thursday 1st August 1996

Felt fine even took the boys on a trip to Stockley working farm.
(I drove there without any problems, the boys loved seeing the animals and riding on a tractor. However I felt as though I was being tested, as there was a woman who stood in front of no2 son blocking his view to seeing a horse being shod, I had a word with her and her reply was 'it's tough'. I felt very angry and stifling this anger made me upset as though I wasn't sticking up for my children properly. I must say however that I think that I handled the situation appropriately and thought to myself that the other woman just wasn't a nice person and I felt pleased that I didn't lower myself to her level).

Friday 2nd July (3rd day on Depixol injection)

AM-felt nervous, legs twitching, however, no disturbing thoughts. I just keep smelling the bad smell from the farm yesterday.

PM-feel brilliant, I've been on a shopping spree and I have got into a size 10 outfit- now I've got to go out!

Annie Moon

Saturday 3rd of August 1996 (4th day on depixol)

I went out last night, I had a lovely time. I had no odd thoughts and I was OK with the crowds.

This morning I though for a moment that there was radioactive fall out dust on the leaves of the trees- I just told myself to pull myself together!

I think now and again, not all the time-, the thought just comes into my head that everything will be alright now that the toybox has gone and the spirit of the dead body has gone with it.

PM
Feeling smashing, listening to music. I've ironed, washed up and put clothes away- we are going camping tomorrow and I am really looking forward to it.

Monday 5th August 1996 (6th day on Depixol)

I was walking on the beach when I saw an impression in the sand, I felt very nervous as if it was a sign of 'Black Magic'. I was alright once I'd destroyed it.

(I thought that I was well at the time of going camping, however I do remember going through

TO SCHIZOPHRENIA AND BACK

the motions of taking care of the boys and cooking etc. I felt as though I was an animation, existing. I tried to feel normal by calling my children 'love' all the time. This verbal act, I felt, was masking the fact that I felt as though I was floating and on autopilot. The fact that every other word to my children was an 'out of character' term of affection, as I always call them 'sweetheart, babes or darling', really irritated my husband to the point of him asking me to stop saying it. It was then I knew I wasn't fooling anybody).

(The sign of black magic really frightened me, it was on a secluded beach- how could it have gotten there, there was nobody about, I felt as though it was a bad sign)

Tuesday 6th August 1996 (7th day on Depixol)

I felt ok today, however I want to close my eyes every time I want to sit down.

Wednesday 7th August 1996 (8th day on Depixol)

I felt tired and twitchy. My legs are restless, I shake constantly, I can understand the distress someone must feel who suffers from Parkinson's disease.

Annie Moon

Thursday 8th August 1996 (9th day on depixol)

Feel fine, legs twitching. I don't want to go to sleep every 5 minutes. (*Twitching makes me look as though I am really nervous about something or that I am on drugs i.e. illegal substances, which I am most definitely not. Friends have also commented. The whole business is very unpleasant*)

Friday 9th August 1996 (10th day on Depixol)

Feel very well, no thoughts, wide awake, restless-(bored). I have done the ironing hoovering and shopping. I wish that I could feel like this all the time- my legs aren't twitching so much either.

2 Weeks later
The witching, anxiety, tiredness were all taking their toll on me. I decided to stop the constant injection of depixol and start back on the chlorpromazine.

TO SCHIZOPHRENIA AND BACK

Friday ? 29th August 1996

Felt brilliant all week still taking chlorpromazine, it's no big deal anymore. My side effects are a dry mouth, dizziness on standing and weight gain.

I feel very positive towards my future now that I have enrolled at college.

2 YEARS LATER
Saturday 14th November 1998 1215pm

Am I a clairvoyant I wonder, hearing the voices of the dead? I saw a spirit of a man at football practice.

Toddy said to increase my risperidone to 16mg so I did as well as taking 5mg droperidol. I feel that my liver is being poisoned and that I am a clairvoyant and it should take its course.

I don't feel sad, I feel ok. I am sorry if I have upset Toddy. We are going to buy me 2 new c.d.s later and a few bits and bobs.

Annie Moon

3 months later
Saturday 27th February 1999

I feel like I want to be alone. I just want to drive to the reservoir and stay there for a while. I keep feeling that there are cameras everywhere watching me and plotting against me. I feel that eye contact will transfer my soul. I saw two identical cars one behind the other and thought that it meant something special to me, yet I don't know what, as if it was some kind of omen- good or bad, I don't know, maybe death.

Its all my own fault that I think these things. I've been trying to manage on 5mg a week of olanzapine, instead of the 10-20mg that I normally take. I feel that life is not for me. I feel that I have spent so much energy on battling with my thoughts that I am now tired and I just want a rest.

I feel that people- maybe the police -are listening in on my telephone calls.

I am not depressed, just tired of it all. The voices in my head are full of conflict: - 'don't trust her, don't look at him', 'she thinks you're after her husband because you smiled'. 'You look like a lesbian, all the children think so'.

I feel so vulnerable and pathetic. I phoned my CPN (community psychiatric nurse), but I felt like an attention seeker and a time waster.

TO SCHIZOPHRENIA AND BACK

Sunday 28th February 1999

God is punishing me.

Monday 29th February 1999

Leave me alone. They're all listening!

I know that you are trying to get into my mind, but I won't let you. I want help, but **SHE** won't let me.

Thursday 4th March 1999

Felt quite low today.

Friday 5th March 1999 1pm

I have taken 20mg olanzapine for nearly 5 days. I feel a lot better. I went to Ruth's this morning and I saw a man lighting a cigarette- I thought he was talking on a radio to the police. I also thought that I saw my birth mother in the post office. I don't feel too suspicious, although I think that people are talking badly about me. I do feel much better.

Annie Moon

1320hrs

Just thinking about my birth mother, she lives out of town and has come to my town to torment me!!

1 YEAR LATER

Friday 2nd June 2000

Here are experiences over the last week, while they are still fresh in my mind.

I had been so well for 9 weeks not taking any tablets. I became like a spirit occupying a human body that didn't belong to me. My limbs seemed so complicated with their blood supply, nerves, bones and muscles- I felt that even if my arm was chopped off I wouldn't feel it. I went down town it was always busy, it always is. I felt like I was floating and everyone was looking at me knowing that I wasn't part of their human race. The spirits told me that they will come and get me back when they are ready- I don't recognise their faces- I looked at old photographs to see if I could recognise them but I couldn't. They tell me that there is a camera and a microphone in the speaker on the living room wall, put there to observe my movements like in the film 'The Truman Show'. They say that my speech will go and that I will die on the tablets and my soul- well

TO SCHIZOPHRENIA AND BACK

that's another story. I can't- couldn't answer the phone because it was a land line and people were listening in.

Toddy phoned the CPN, I don't really know why, I think maybe he was concerned that I couldn't or didn't want to communicate with the human race. I felt trapped and scared that the CPN will have my children taken away from me and scared that they will put me in hospital where I will die. I felt so trapped that I agreed to take some tablets rather than talk to him.

The next day 2 people came and I was even more anxious that there was a trap- why 2 people? Is one a social worker?

The spirits told me that Toddy wanted me dead- I couldn't sleep for a week for fear that he would smother me- I felt powerless to do anything. I would never harm anybody except in self defence. I carried a knife around with me for a while, while I felt weird- something which now frightens me.

The spirits watched and made comments while we were in bed having sex. They did not say anything derogatory- I can't remember what they said, but they weren't nasty. I felt that they were my allies.

Things were suddenly made clear this evening, I

Annie Moon

will take as much medicine as it takes to feel safe and secure. I do love my family.

The medicine makes me feel better- not so suspicious- I just hope that these feelings don't come back.

I felt spirits touching me at times- only on the arm or on my back. I saw shadows, heard bangs and footsteps, knocks and spirits at the window. My head ached, my eyes were dry, I felt nauseous at times, I had no appetite, I was thirsty and all I could do was listen to the rhythm of the music.

I hope that this is it and the spirits won't summon me.

Monday 13th October 2003 11.30pm

I cannot remember much about today, except that I had to go to town. I went on the bus, smells were acute. I was clean and smart. I checked my bank balance and I don't know where all my money has gone. All the time I felt that I was being watched, every window that I looked in I felt that a third party was noting down what I was looking at. All day I have been constantly snacking on biscuits. My period started this pm. This morning my stomach was sore and my throat/voice box was 'dusty'. I think that it was the Pariet for indigestion- I won't take it tonight. I have felt sad today- not depressed, but I have felt that

TO SCHIZOPHRENIA AND BACK

music affects my brain pattern and I feel that the sad suicidal thoughts need to be walked off. I thought that I will do that tomorrow by walking to the reservoir whilst the boys are at school. I don't feel physically or mentally with depression- in fact one minute I might have plans of writing down ideas of learning the guitar, reading and doing my cross-stitch. I have slept these last 2 nights with the help of 5mg Stilnoct and 1mg of Lorazepam. I phoned the chemist to see if my medicine was ready, it wasn't. I feel that I want to be isolated- I feel that I have no conversation in me that I want to share. I love my Todd and the boys but I feel that he is looking out for signs of illness all the time. I crossed the road outside the building society to avoid a tramp, I thought that I heard him wolf whistle and mutter something. I trod on a coca cola can in the street and fell over onto my knees, I was upset at bringing more attention to myself, my 'scanning' became more acute as I waited for the bus home in the bus station. My knees were sore but ok. I phoned Todd (and was upset) - to cancel badminton. I then broke my toe by opening a door on it at home. I did the tea and fed the boys and No 2 son's friend O. I washed up and put washing on the maiden. I like it when the kids are about. When I was alone again, I wanted to buy a new Walkman for tomorrow. I have no plans to die just thoughts. I feel that if I keep walking, God will give me a voice or a sign be it from him or spirits. I feel that people are

Annie Moon

looking in at the window. I hear knocking and tapping when there's nobody there. I hear my name being called. I cancelled my appointment with A the psychiatric social worker for tomorrow. I am supposed to be seeing B but I want to be alone with my thoughts. I am never bored; I have too many things going through my mind. I have decided to write down what I am thinking, if I can remember.

The last couple of days, I have taken Quetiapine 450mg. I feel that people don't believe me, nobody listens and when I do explain, they form opinions about me, they think that I am an attention seeker. I wouldn't bother anybody if I really thought at times that I could do it alone.

Somebody once told me, write your feelings down on paper, they can't judge and won't answer back.

I have been so upset that I have cried for all the victims of schizophrenia, whose lives have been taken out of their control and their worlds turned upside down.

In moments where I don't have thoughts and pictures in my mind of jumping off a motorway bridge or meeting the 'Lady of the Lake', I have thought about how I could help other people. Give myself a purpose, help to give shelter and warmth to those who are suffering with the terrible thoughts, voices, smells, touches. I know what its like to be cold and I know what its like to be in

TO SCHIZOPHRENIA AND BACK

hospital where you are locked in. Sometimes it's far more dangerous for me to be in hospital than it is for me to be wandering about on the moors and the streets, with the drunks and the junkies.

Some people in hospital treat you with no human rights. I would prefer to be in a prison cell-'talk to me', yes talk and you will get some **more** Lorazepam- become **more** suicidal and become **more** of an attention seeker. I think of helping others and then not.

I wrote the words to a song down once and my Mum went weird on me as if I was writing down my own words- I was about 10 years old at the time, I really wish I could remember the song.

I've thought about arranging my own funeral, not out of morbidity, but out of practicality. I know that the only people to miss me will be my boys. I don't want to be like Nobby, without a headstone. I feel that if I am buried, God will have me buried alive.

I have been thinking a lot about my Nana, things have come to my attention through physical occurrences and dreams and thoughts. I feel that she and Nobby were with me at Piccadilly train station last week- that's when I felt calm and invincible and that I wanted to be back with my family because I knew it would be ok.

Annie Moon

It's like when I went to the moors a while ago, I lay down to die and out of nowhere came runners and out of nowhere came a 'golf ball' sized hailstone- another message from God.

I snapped at Todd earlier, I was after an exercise book to write my thoughts down in and he asked me why I wanted an exercise book. I said 'what do you normally use them for?' I didn't want to share the fact that I would rather write down my thoughts in a book than speak to anybody.

Goodnight love Annie X

12am I do not have any suicidal thoughts at this moment

A CPN telephoned, I was afraid of speaking to her.

Wednesday 16th October 2003 0900hrs

Didn't hardly sleep last night, I had a night sweat. When I did sleep, I dreamt and the dreams woke me up. I woke up feeling happy and motivated. I took 150mg of Quetiapine, it calmed me down a bit. I have had thoughts that Toddy doesn't really want me around except for my financial contribution. I keep the house spotless, clothes ironed and washed and he never comments. He never ever asks me what I've done during the day,

TO SCHIZOPHRENIA AND BACK

 or who I've spoken to. If I don't initiate conversation- we wouldn't have any at all. He tells me frequently that he's planning for a life with just him and the boys and that he plans his finances to that effect. He often says when I come out of hospital that he would give me a lump sum and that I can give him a set amount to look after the boys. I feel worthless at times- but I tell you what- it makes me more determined to do the things that I want to do for myself e.g. my university course. Why should I do what he says e.g. have long hair etc when he doesn't respect me or love me and when the kids are older, won't even be with me. I have no desire for another partner or house or children, I am very content. He sighs or moans when the kids need anything buying e.g. No 2 needing a school jumper. He sulks for days if he has to spend money. He said to me the other day that the monetary cost of the conservatory could have been used for him and the boys to live off for a few years. He ignores me when I am on a period- he doesn't sleep and certainly lets me know about it, he huffs and puffs and sighs all the time_ it is certainly helping me to write this down. He sulks if he doesn't get sex. He rewards me with conversation if we do have sex.

I am determined to be strong and healthy, both mentally and physically. I will come out of this o.k., I love my boys. I love Toddy. I try and imagine seeing the faces of other fanciable men when we have sex, but I can't orgasm unless I see Toddy. He has gradually taken over and it feels that he is slowly doing without me. It feels that he is trying to be a single parent- I'm with the boys most of the time and I hug, talk to and look after them, but when Toddy is here my role is redundant, it's as if he is creating a competition of who is the better parent e.g. No 2 son is his sidekick. No 2 son lies in bed with me, we go places and do things in the holidays e.g. fishing and swimming, bike riding and walking. But Toddy says to him that <u>he'll</u> always be there for him- <u>there</u>, I've got it off my chest now!

I don't feel like mixing today except to go to the gym and maybe Piccadilly train station to get a refund on my Blackpool ticket. I need to get No 2 son a school jumper. My back is still sore at about the 5th thoracic vertebrate, despite going to the gym.

0930

Returned CPN's call, I left my name- she was not in the office.

1455

Got home from the gym and getting No2's jumper at Tescos, there was a message from CPN regarding a visit. There was a message regarding

TO SCHIZOPHRENIA AND BACK

my contact lenses. I don't feel like talking to anybody, but my mood is o.k. since exercising. There was a funny thing when I got home- there was a bag of crisps on the work surface instead of on top of the cupboards- has somebody been home? There were no signs of shoes etc from Toddy or the boys. Is it a sign, or is it Mr Jingles the mouse? What is going on? The bus driver was very jolly, he made me smile. I just feel like writing, writing, writing, my best friend.

I found out that the crisps were from No 1 son coming home during the day for his P.E kit.

1530

Feeling low, I have been listening to a music channel on SKY television, the music gives my thoughts rhythm- I am starting some of my customers' ironing.

Cooked tea, I feel that if I concentrate on the kids and keeping a clean house that I can get by.

2233

I feel that Toddy knows every thought that I am writing. I suspect that he goes through my things

Annie Moon

when I am out of the room. He has given me no conversation this evening. I cooked his tea and made him a couple of drinks, then spent the night in No1's room watching T.V with No2. I am managing if people don't pressure me. He was watching football, (*He meaning Toddy*). I felt like going walking with my pyjamas on, took 300mg quetiapine, it has helped to stop my jaw feeling tight.

Todd is in bed, I've got my bedside light on- he is sighing making a point.

Physically, my back hurts when I cough, and my nose is a bit runny, but mentally, I feel that I am keeping it together- I feel weepy at times, but I won't give in- I won't leave the boys and I won't be pushed out of my own home. The boys are my life and I want them to know that they are loved- I want them to be strong healthy young men with good happy lives.

The boys and me are supposed to be going to the Isle of Man in a week's time, but I can't bring myself to speak to my Dad and step mum but I want to take the boys to see them. I don't want to communicate, I need to concentrate and focus on doing a good job as a mum- I don't feel sad at the moment, in fact I just want a cup of tea.

At times I feel that I am omnipresent. I feel that if I don't look at somebody, then they can't see me (*as if I was invisible*). I feel that if I do look at

TO SCHIZOPHRENIA AND BACK

someone then they know what I am thinking and they know all about me and that they are taking notes, (*as if they were big brother*). I feel like running off my thoughts by physically running tomorrow- I'll see.

I feel that the spirits are present and are keeping me strong.

Dear God keep my family safe tonight, thank you Annie XXX

I want to get my book looked at but I feel such need for my own isolation that I'd rather not. I feel that people don't think I'm safe around my kids but I am, I'm a good mum.

2300hrs

I feel tired now- I'll pass on the brew and try and get some sleep!

Thursday 17th October 2003

Took 150mg quetiapine.

Todd is still ignoring me. I know that he doesn't want me around. I couldn't breathe last night because of a cold; he never asked if I was alright. He didn't even report me missing the other week for 3 days and then he only reported me missing because No 1 son was worried and upset.

Even though I love my house I will look for somewhere else; I know that the boys won't be living with me full time but they will have their own bedrooms and can treat it as their second home. Toddy always says that I wouldn't be able to survive on my own, that I wouldn't be able to cope.

He has said in the past that if we split up then he will move away. I feel that I should stay for the sake of the boys but I feel that I have had my life sucked out of me and that can't be good for them.

Toddy is always going on about his friends who are single parents. I feel that he always likes to be a martyr.

He never commented on my hair cut, he always says that I could never look like the woman he married.
I feel mentally tired.

Picked up contact lenses and went for a refund on my train ticket.

<u>Thursday afternoon</u>

Looked at houses and phoned Todd up to arrange

TO SCHIZOPHRENIA AND BACK

a financial settlement. I will be around the corner (*in my new house*). I feel zingy, floaty, liquidy and I swear I feel hypoglycaemic despite eating.

Todd came home at the usual time, we talked for hours. I had a headache and my eyes and back hurt- I gradually came out of my 'mood', 'state of mind', and I realised that I hadn't been myself recently. I was upset, irritable and irrational.

I took quetiapine 350mg, (*antipsychotic*), lorazepam 1mg, (*for anxiety)* and 5mg of stilnoct to help me to sleep. We are ok again.

I told him that I wanted £65,000 pounds; he could have everything, even the clothes pegs and plants. I would be living around the corner, the boys could come and go as they pleased, I will still do all their ironing and I will still look after the boys after school and in the holidays and at weekends.

We spoke, I felt that I needed to get away, go to a hotel. I felt the need for isolation. I don't want to have to face my step mum and dad in the I.O.M, I'd rather just take me and the boys somewhere- we'll see. I managed to stay at home despite being 'stressed'.

We cuddled etc and I felt that a switch had been turned off.

Annie Moon

I not only chose a house, but I wrote down all the furniture and equipment that I would need. I am so sorry that I upset Toddy but I felt that I wanted isolation so much and I didn't want to be cold again (*i.e. sitting on the moors in freezing temperatures*).

Toddy cried, he says that he only cares about me and the boys. He says that he can tell when I am ill and just steers clear of me because if he does ask how I am, I bite his head off because of my paranoia- it is at these times that I think that he wants to put me away. He says far from it, he would rather I tell him what the matter is, then he can help me. Sometimes I don't realize how nasty I can be until after I've taken my medication.

Todd says he knows when I'm not myself, because I sit in the television chair staring out of the window, (*I am what I call scanning i.e. observing every minute visible detail of people, objects and noises*) and moving my head as if I was talking to somebody in my head, he says that then I look around the living room to see if I'm being watched. He is right, I am.

Friday 18th October 2004

Took quetiapine 200mg. Woke up in a good mood- feel hypoglycaemic, back sore. Phoned my G.P, they were taking emergencies only- I will phone again on Monday if mentally o.k. Head

TO SCHIZOPHRENIA AND BACK

feels floaty, feeling a bit 'zingy', but relaxing. I phoned the rehab team- ? Somebody is coming at 3pm.

<u>A message came from God through the television:</u> those who believe in the Lord will have eternity in Heaven. Those who believe will have an eternal life. The Lord giveth and the Lord taketh away. You come into this world with nothing and you leave it with nothing. Blessed are the meek for they shall inherit the earth.

I have a headache, 'embers' behind my eyes, took 2 paracetamol- (not like me) like burning electric wires…..Go to the gym.

I feel like I need to be anaesthetised for a couple of weeks in a cupboard.

Next door drilling again!

I thought that I was the one who stank at the gym.

<u>1220hrs</u>

got back from the gym- messages on the phone- J for ironing, (a little job that helps to keep me sane), the upholsterers and my C.P.N. cancelled his visit- I feel some relief- maybe I should just keep my thoughts private- I'd rather sit on the moors than have my thoughts discussed as childish or nonsense or attention seeking which I feel my C.P.N thinks.

I feel upset thinking these thoughts; my mind doesn't want to switch off. I have thought after thought- I think too much! I took 50mg of quetiapine. I felt like I was being watched whilst I was out, and that the women at the gym were undercover. I just focused on the music on the television whilst I exercised- I know there is nothing that I can do about them- I enjoyed the gym. I must make sure that I am not chunnerring aloud to myself in the steam room and the sauna as I feel that they have hidden cameras there.

My mood is o.k.

1505 hrs

Scanning

I am feeling 'nicer' as a person since taking my medication. I feel that if someone came to the door, then I could answer it and have a brief polite conversation- something that I couldn't have done earlier today.

1520

I can't seem to watch television programmes, I just keep flicking through the channels- I feel better

TO SCHIZOPHRENIA AND BACK

with the music channels giving my mind and my thoughts some rhythm.

Zypexa was a far better medicine for my mind, if it weren't for the 4 stones weight gain, which is coming off now that I've changed medicines.

1530
I feel sad

1545

I feel o.k. but my head feels 'zingy'. I wanted to speak to my G.P. but he's away until Monday. I feel like my head is going to explode. I rang my C.P.N to see if I could go back on zyprexa- he said that he will send another C.P.N to ring me tomorrow. I took 150mg of quetiapine and 2mg of lorazepam, ate some tea, nervously/ hurriedly. I can feel my head is going 'muzzy' and shutting down. I fell asleep at 5.30pm.

1945

Wow! I didn't know where I was or what day it was when I woke up, but I feel great, I am in an excellent mood.

Felt great all evening, I want more of this feeling- I still have brain ache from thinking

Annie Moon

2250

I took 200mg of quetiapine, 1mg of lorazepam and 5mg of stilnoct. <u>Slept really well</u>

Saturday 19th October 2003

0900

I took 200mg of quetiapine, my mood is really good. Minds thoughts won't let up- nothing unpleasant. I keep hearing tapping at the window and knocking at the door all day. My head is tired from all the thoughts and medication! I feel like taking a nap.

I keep walking into things as if I were drunk

1030

I keep smelling faeces on me- I can't pinpoint it but I keep getting pockets (wafts) of it. I thought that I could hear the helicopters and the jets in the sky.

1300

I feel smashing- Dad telephoned me and left a message whilst I was out and I answered it when I felt ready. My step mum asked me where I was when they rang, I said that I was pegging washing out- I am looking forwards to going to the Isle of

TO SCHIZOPHRENIA AND BACK

Man to see them next weekend. At this moment in time, I wish that the gym was open and I could work out. I think that I might go for a walk. I know that my step mum looks out for my Dad but I really don't wish for them to worry- I love them both and I feel ashamed to even talk about any of the events occurring due to the schizophrenia. It took me years to stop thinking that they thought I am a drama queen- attention seeker; in fact, I just <u>don't</u> talk about it to them.

<u>1400</u>

I relaxed whilst listening to music in the conservatory. I tried phoning Phoebe to see if she fancied a walk, she was out so I left a message on the answer machine.

<u>1500</u>

My head is aching with too much thinking. I'll make tea and when everybody's doing their thing I'll dose myself up and go to bed- oh not to think for 2 weeks!

Spoke to Dad today, people are listening in! C.P.N rang and she is coming tomorrow morning

<u>Bed Time</u>

Annie Moon

300mg quetiapine, 1mg lorazepam, 5mg stilnoct

Relaxed with brain ache ------------------------
Annie
___

Went on the schizophrenia chat room site on the internet to ask about 'scanning' and to see what people had to say about the drugs. The way that things appeared was that people put on a vast amount of weight with their drugs.

Phoebe phoned, it was lovely to speak to her- I felt o.k. I did think that somebody might have the phone tapped- I didn't say anything incriminating. I haven't a clue what we talked about!

Sunday 20th October 2003

0800

I went in the schizophrenia chat room for information on zyprexa- everyone on this drug has put vast amounts of weight on- I've just realised that I've already written this! I do sometimes think that I never had as many suicidal thoughts whilst taking olanzapine (zyprexa). I feel that I may not have been on the internet- it feels like a dream. Just like the 'real thought dream' that I had when I thought that I'd picked the boys up from primary school whilst I was topless- it took months to convince me that I didn't do it.

TO SCHIZOPHRENIA AND BACK

0845

I took 200mg quetiapine. Slept well, I woke up and did the washing, drying and cleaned the kitchen before I got washed and dressed. My eyes feel like they are staring, for example exophthalmos that you get with a goitre or overactive thyroid gland- maybe that's why they burn behind them- too much staring and thinking- my optician says that my eyes are healthy except for poor vision. I don't think for one minute that I've actually <u>got</u> exopthalmos, it just feels like it.

I'm in a good mood.

<u>Today's plans</u>

A C.P.N is coming from the rehabilitation team; I'm going to go to the gym; Todd and I are going to go and choose some wallpaper for the bedroom. I'm going to do our ironing and J's ironing.

On a scale of 1 to 10 my brain ache is a **2** at this moment in time.

0905

Feeling light headed and wobbly.

Annie Moon

0930

I feel confused at times, I can't think properly e.g. a full sentence in one go. Looking in drawers and not the c.d. rack for c.d.s. I am listening to music in the conservatory, to give my brain a rhythm and to close my eyes.

I sometimes wonder if this pain in my back is caused by an inhaled contact lens. I have swallowed one once but I can't remember inhaling one. Or it could be a piece of sweet corn.

Psychic premonition xxxxx carries a knife under the seat of her car!!!!

The music's rhythm and words stop you thinking on thoughts so much- you tend to concentrate on the lyrics and the beat.

The C.P.N has been and I don't know what she has said!

Brain ache **4**

I rested in bed for half an hour to help my brain ache. When up my head is full of unconnected, unrelated, random crappy thoughts.

1pm

Todd's come home from work. I can smell solvents in the front room.

TO SCHIZOPHRENIA AND BACK

I went up to the D.I.Y store with Todd and No 2, I felt weird, surreal and liquidy. Brain ache **7,** I took 2 paracetamol. All is o.k., it has been nice and quiet this afternoon.
Went on the chat room site to see if anybody has answered my question on 'scanning'- not a single answer! Is it work from the devil? He is putting thoughts into my head- I am for safety's sake not putting down my every thought on paper- I am not evil and if necessary, I will sleep at the gates of heaven.

Didn't go to the gym, I felt tired and I didn't want to do J's ironing, I will do it tomorrow. I want to get my back looked at soon, but I don't want to put my safety in jeopardy by going to the doctors. I have just taken 400mg of quetiapine. I will not take any others, however, I will take them tomorrow if I can't sleep.

Did my own ironing, the creases seem impossible to get out tonight. I feel very smelly.

My mood is quite stable. I keep going hot and cold. I just want peace and quiet tomorrow. Good night, God bless my family, I wish them healthy, happy lives. Xxx

I love my boys.

Annie Moon

Plans for the I.O.M are walk, walk and more walking.

I fancy learning the guitar. I have a terrible piano pitch/ electricity noise in my ears from the outside.

0800hrs Monday 21st October 2003

I didn't sleep too well last night; I had night terrors whilst I was awake. I thought that somebody was in the house and they were going to batter us all with a baseball bat- I kept saying to myself as I was frozen with fear that the only way they could get in would be through the kitchen window as it has an outside seal on the u.p.v.c. I had night sweats.

0845

I made an appointment to see my G.P regarding my back. I don't really want to go but I feel that I have an abscess in my back inside, due to something being inhaled.

It's funny, but I've not had heartburn for a while… not that I can remember anyway.

Brain ache **2,** took 200mg quetiapine.

0930

Listening to 60's music puts me in a good mood.

TO SCHIZOPHRENIA AND BACK

1020

Brain ache **0** – I think that it is because I've been to the toilet. I have music playing inside my head- My CPN Streisand. I know when I smell- I can read others thoughts and what they think.

1050

I feel anxious and my mouth is dry.

1100

My G.P. checked my back-I have not inhaled anything, he offered some physiotherapy- I declined. (*Unbeknown to me he rang my C.P.N. out of concern for my mental well being*).

1145

I have indigestion- I have taken water and an antacid. I am listening to music on Sky TFM. My mood is o.k. I've got to do J's ironing.

2.30pm

Did J's ironing; I found £10 in the pockets <u>again</u>!

Annie Moon

Is she testing my honesty? Bad thoughts- can't write them down, but I would rather be in isolation on the moors.

I feel sad on occasions, I am <u>NOT</u> depressed. I feel like walking until the bad thoughts go and the good thoughts come.

Listening to music puts sounds, rhythm and words in my head, leaving little room for unwanted thoughts and sounds- the rhythm affects my mood, yet Celine Dion etc is relaxing- <u>NOT</u> depressing.

I keep hearing taps, knocks and sounds on the doors, windows and upstairs.

MUSIC MUSIC MUSIC MUSIC MUSIC MUSIC MUSIC MUSIC MUSIC MUSIC MUSIC MUSIC MUSIC MUSIC MUSIC MUSIC
!!
!!
!!!!

<u>2.50pm</u>

I keep smelling sweaty feet- I used some air freshener.

<u>2.55pm</u>

Starting to 'scan', wanting to walk it off.

TO SCHIZOPHRENIA AND BACK

3.30pm

I cut No 1's hair, my mood is o.k. I just feel like I'm floating all the time. I cooked tea.

I noted some writing on No 2's school diary, when I asked about it to No2, he said that I wrote it this morning. I couldn't remember and I couldn't work out what it said?!#

6.15pm

I just want to go to sleep- to be anaesthetised for a while to make me feel better. I feel that my mind is in torment, I have no spare room for outside thoughts and conversation. Mood o.k. took quetiapine 400mg, 1mg lorazepam. I will take a sleeping tablet if I need to.

Mood absolutely fine, did tea, washed up and hovered.

I still don't want to speak to anybody. I must hide this book whilst I am asleep, it is <u>very private.</u> I feel fine and content seeing Todd and the boys today, I love them very much.
I accidentally spilt boiling water on my leg whilst draining the potatoes at tea time.

Annie Moon

9.30pm

I have felt smashing since the medication has taken effect, only heard the knocking and the doorbell a couple of times when my mind was playing tricks on me. I'd feel more sociable if someone were to phone up. Helped No 2 with his homework- I am taking 5mg stilnoct to help with my sleep.

Tuesday 22nd October 2003

0700

Slept well, woke up a few times but I don't have any lasting damage from my dreams. I feel very well this morning, happy and motivated. I am going to the gym later. B is dropping his ironing off later, cleaned around this morning.

0800

Took 250mg quetiapine- I feel 'drunk', I fancy watching Kilroy on television rather than listening to music.

0915

Hearing the doorbell again! Nobody is there. Sometimes I feel that my heart misses a beat. I feel very relaxed. Light headed when I stand up. I can hear my heart and I can feel the blood

TO SCHIZOPHRENIA AND BACK

pumping through my veins- I need to lie down.

<u>0940</u>

Banged into a door and bruised my hip- I am writing this in case I die so it will explain my bruises.

I rang my C.P.N. She is not in, a message was left for her to call me later.

<u>1000</u>

My C.P.N rang back and offered a visit. I feel all defensive, antisocial and suspicious. I want to be isolated except for being with Toddy and the boys.

I can smell urine in the front room and on me.

<u>1045</u>

I went to the building society and the bank in town. I felt like I was being followed and watched.

Went to the gym and worked off my thoughts, I was slightly paranoid in the gym, but it's always very quiet when I go. Felt sad at times. Scanning.

Annie Moon

12pm

Message from school re: No 1 son- he has walked out of school and not handed his coursework in- he had told me that he had done it and that it was at school.

4pm

I am paranoid and irritable.

5pm

I fancy a run and I want to teach myself the guitar. The message from school must have been a mistake- No 1's report has been signed by all his teachers and his work is being handed in tomorrow as suggested by the teacher.
No 2 had some unwelcome comments in his school diary- which is not like him- he and his friend say that another boy was causing trouble and the boys mum actually apologised to No 2 after school.

5.10pm

I feel fine, took quetiapine 100mg

6pm

Scanning and paranoid, I feel like a walk, I need to get away for a while. Hearing noises on the stairs-

TO SCHIZOPHRENIA AND BACK

I can hear knocks on the doors and windows. My mood is o.k.

7.30pm

I think that I've annoyed Todd, (he thought it was funny). Tonight for tea I cooked what I thought were pork chops, so I cooked them in a sweet and sour sauce served with rice- they were in fact lamb chops- I <u>thought</u> they were fatty! Todd said that it was the first time that he'd ever had sweet 'n' sour lamb and that he was in fact looking forward to lamb with mint sauce on them. I thought that I'd cooked a lovely tea for everybody.

9.15pm

I have enjoyed my time with No 2 son this evening. I have a headache. I am anxious about my son at school. Took quetiapine 250mg. I thought that it was snowing earlier, but it was my mind playing tricks again.

My thoughts on keeping a diary now

I don't keep a diary anymore as reading it after recovering from a psychotic episode is very upsetting. Also since going back on Zyprexa (Olanzapine) I have on the whole been functioning very well.

Hospital admissions

There have been several. Mainly involuntary admissions where the police have taken me to the hospital because I have put myself at risk by wandering the streets at night or walking to lonely stretches of the moors with suicidal ideas. However the many times that I have done this, I have not felt depressed, more a feeling of calmness and invincibility. I would go to the moors and challenge God by saying, 'if you want me then take me!' I remember one night that I was up there on the moors, on my 'bench in the sky', when it was very late and extremely dark. It started hail stoning giant balls of ice; this was after I'd challenged God. I thought it was his way of saying 'go home you stupid woman!' The hail stones would have caused serious injury as well as hypothermia.

On a few occasions a psychiatric worker would quiz me about what it was like to hallucinate, as he had spent thousands of pounds over the years on drugs trying to recreate experiences like mine- I did feel at one point, (never having taken drugs except in the case of a bun my brother fed me which contained marihuana when I was fourteen), that I was quite fortunate that I was getting it all for free!!! Of course this is a stupid notion and I can see why when people are psychotic they would turn to street drugs and alcohol to try to feel some

TO SCHIZOPHRENIA AND BACK

sense of normality.

On one occasion I remember my consultant knocking on my front door. I thought she was a visiting Jehovah's Witness. I remember thinking why is Dr S coming to convert me.

During this episode I thought that two thousand souls from the 9/11 terrorist attack on New York were in my carpet. My carpet has tiny flowers in it and each one was a spirit. I wanted to join them all up with some cello tape but I didn't have any available, so I lit dozens of candles and placed them on the floor in what unwittingly turned out to be in the Jewish Star of David.

Of course I was admitted and despite being against the admission and the holding me down in hospital for injections, I was glad to get better to say the least!

During a couple of episodes, of which there have been many, two comments that have been made have really affected me. They are 'you're acting child like' and 'you're playing with me'. These were both made by professionals when I was ill.

Of course this doesn't help to encourage one to communicate for fear of ridicule or rejection as on many occasions I would be paranoid anyway and would feel that people were laughing at me. I am

Annie Moon

putting these incidents in my book for these professionals as they will know who they are and maybe it will improve things for the next patient.

I did suffer with reactionary depression during the early days of my illness. This felt far worse mentally than any psychosis that I have had. Yet it wasn't treated with as much urgency. I really feel for those people who suffer with depression and I would definitely rather be 'mad' than depressed, going on the feelings that I encountered. Obviously this will differ with different people.

TO SCHIZOPHRENIA AND BACK

CHAPTER SIX

RECOVERY

I have received lots of help from lots of different people most of whom are listed below

- Community Psychiatric Nurses (CPNs)
- Police
- Consultant Psychiatrists
- Support Workers
- Day Hospital
- Family Doctor
- Clinical Psychologist
- Family
- Friends

The first input from the CPNs was when I was very unwell in hospital. I had lots of negative symptoms of the schizophrenia such as lack of motivation to do the simplest of things such as washing and dressing.

The CPN would visit my home very regularly. I would feel that I was a fraud and that there were other people who needed her help more than me. I would always ask if she had enough time to see me and say that it was O.K if she wanted to cancel. She very assertively said that she would decide when and for how long our visits would last. This took the pressure of guilt off me by alleviating the thought that there were more deserving, needy people in need of her help.

The CPN would often, in the early days, assess my mental health by using a questionnaire.

The CPN helped by listening and offering ways to change my thoughts and behaviour. I used to get up in the morning, take the children to school and to playgroup. Then I would lie on the settee all day in and out of sleep, feeling very anxious about the simple things such as washing up the pots. My memory was shocking and still is. I have to keep a diary with things that I have to do in it.

I would get off the settee later on in the day to pick the children up and cook tea. My husband used to comment on the food by referring to my meals as 'concoctions', as I would try to make healthy, well balanced meals and yet sometimes they would be bizarre combinations such as those a pregnant woman might crave for! My CPN reassured me that I was trying my best and doing well to even have a meal ready for everybody come meal time.

My CPN involved the help of a Support Worker. The Support Worker was a God send. She would take me shopping, listen to me, offer peer support as she was of a similar age to me. We even went to aerobics. She even came with me to drive a new car that we had bought, as I was apprehensive about driving it.

TO SCHIZOPHRENIA AND BACK

At one point I couldn't get up off the settee and the CPN and the Support Worker came round. I couldn't even motivate myself to get a drink of water. The housework was building up around me and I expressed how anxious and upset I was about the state of the house; they offered to help me clean it. I was so touched that I declined their offer and got off my backside to do it myself.

I realised that to relieve anxiety, I had to tackle small things head on, such as washing up, cooking and cleaning. I soon realised that I gained a sense of achievement from completing tasks/chores. I would write down in a diary, things that I had to do, such as dress the children, walk to school, wash up and many more chores that I had taken for granted before I had full blown schizophrenia. I would tick the chores off in my diary as I completed them and seeing so many ticks at the end of the day gave me that sense of achievement.

I found that planning things to do in my diary meant that I didn't have to remember them. Even now, with all my coping strategies, I can't remember what I have done over the weekend unless I check in my diary; however I do remember important things from years ago. Also, if friends tell me about hospital appointments or special events, I write these down to remind myself to ask about them when I next see them.

Annie Moon

After a while of input from the Support Worker, I became very paranoid, thinking that she thought negatively about my parenting skills. I do a good job with the boys given my circumstances. It really affected our relationship. I stopped seeing her due to the paranoia but was able to carry on with the good work that she had done with me over the years. I am not paranoid now and I would like to thank her for her help.

My CPN gave me a great deal of support when my brother came to stay as he was homeless, alcoholic and recovering from a serious drug addiction. He was very emaciated and he was jaundiced. He was in fact dying. The CPN tried to get him some help and I helped him find somewhere to live. Something he said about my other brother saying that I was a carbon copy of my mother really annoyed me. I thought why would he say something so hurtful? I stopped seeing him, the next time I did see him, he was laid out dead, in a mortuary's visiting room.

My CPN came with me to view the body. My younger brother and birth mother were there, my brother asked the CPN to leave and offer a bit of dignity to my dead brother, (Little did he know how she'd tried to help him and I!) I hadn't seen my birth mother for over 10 years, since the day that she said she couldn't take my two children out together and that she'd had an abortion because she couldn't look after kids.

TO SCHIZOPHRENIA AND BACK

My birth mother is ever the victim.

My Consultant Psychiatrists have changed over the years; all of them have been helpful and accommodating of my needs and have treated me with respect and dignity.

The Consultant that I have at present has known me for ten years. If I have any problems coping I can contact my CPN or my Consultant Psychiatrist's secretary. I have been given permission to see her when needed should she be able to help. I also am able to communicate via e-mail, which I find very reassuring and which really helps to make me feel that I am not on my own in all of this.

Nowadays I see my CPN about once a month, however she will always come sooner should my husband or I telephone her and there is always somebody at the end of the telephone to help, although I find it hard when unwell to speak with unfamiliar people. On one occasion recently I e-mailed my consultant's secretary with a bizarre note which read:-

"Dr S,
I have to go away. I love my children so I will tell them where I am going when I have sorted something out, maybe Scotland. I am trying to be

responsible and not go to the moors. I took some medicine at the weekend and felt that my husband wanted to stab me and kill me; I felt suicidal, it only happened when I took the medicine. I don't at the moment. I haven't read for six weeks. I've even thought of the new hotel nearby. I'm doing really well. I don't want to have to communicate with anyone except my children. My house is clean. I just want to tell you I will come back when I have some medicine in my system as I will need to sleep. I don't want police to take me to the hospital. I don't want paranoia. I am clean."

I really thought that I was being responsible. As a result of this letter, within the course of an hour, I had a Social Worker and a nurse on my sofa, trying to fathom out what my problem was, if I was safe and if they could help.
In other words the support is there if I need it, which is reassuring.
My CPN at the beginning of my treatment helped me with financial matters. She arranged for a visit to Welfare Rights to assess what benefits I could claim after I had retired from nursing. She filled in complicated lengthy benefit forms for me and arranged for somebody to accompany me to a tribunal when the benefits people said that I couldn't have Disability Living Allowance. This ruling was overturned at the tribunal. I couldn't have helped myself at that time as I was far too unwell what with depixol injections as well as tablets with all the side effects as well as the negative symptoms of the schizophrenia- my limit

TO SCHIZOPHRENIA AND BACK

was to school and back.
This practical help started to pave the way for the management of my schizophrenia. I have come to the conclusion now that it is not something that can be cured (for me anyway) but it is something that can be managed and there are now plenty of good times that stamp out memories of the bad times.
The police have been involved on many occasions, they have always been sympathetic and professional. They have deployed dogs, helicopters and have had to be called away from people glassing each other at the pub to help me.
I remember on one occasion when there must have been six police men and women trying to get me in the hospital; eventually they carried me in- I cringe at the thought.
I have gradually, over time, tried to say to myself that they won't recognise me in the street, as every time I would see a police car etc, for a long while, I would have flashbacks of the embarrassment of being carted off by the police to the hospital- I likened this to post traumatic stress disorder. I would recommend to anybody in a similar position to just remember that the police are very busy people, who are professional and just doing their job, with their own lives to lead and you are not so special that they will be looking out for you on the street so that they can comment or ridicule.
I was referred for CBT (Cognitive Behavioural

Annie Moon

Therapy). The CBT was to change my behaviour and my thinking process during certain situations. It has worked to a certain extent in that now, instead of wandering the streets or the moors, I will book myself into a hotel. I also try my best to let people know where I am going, so long as I don't feel threatened by a hospital admission.

When I first met Dr D, my consultant psychologist, I felt really self-centred talking about me for an hour. He, on the other hand, gave me permission to speak, and offered his approval of my speaking, saying that it was my time.

I disclosed everything to Dr D about my dysfunctional family, illness etc, and I did this early on, at my pace. I felt that if he knew everything, then maybe it would help.

When our sessions ended Dr D said that I could ring him at the office if I needed any more help. I have done this a couple of times when CPNs that I know have not been available. Dr D has been of great support in dealing with life management; I think Dr D is Britain's very own answer to a Dr Phil Mcgraw!!

Now, instead of walking on the moors, I have access -although very limited- to the respite bed.

There is a respite bed; however there is only one bed for a large area of population and this is usually booked up. This, theoretically, would prevent a hospital admission, so long as risk could be managed.

I would recommend that there be better respite facilities as surely this would ultimately reduce the need for hospital beds and their cost.

TO SCHIZOPHRENIA AND BACK

I tried Day Hospital for a very short while. My children were very young at the time and I had no help in looking after them whilst I went to the Day Hospital. Maybe it should be a recommended that there be crèche facilities close by to the hospital so that parents can attend for their therapies. The other thing that I didn't like was that nobody spoke to me- maybe I looked scary with my shakes and fidgeting Parkinson type symptoms (due to medication). Needless to say I must have only attended for three or four sessions.

I was reluctant to go because, when they did a register of the patients attending, my name was not on it, even though my consultant and CPN had arranged it. Little things like this used to set off paranoia; I felt as though I was not welcome, when it was merely a clerical error.

I think what may have helped me, apart from childcare, would have been to have had a personal named nurse who could have introduced one to other people and maybe initiated conversations.

I can initiate conversations now, but this is down to years of reflecting on situations and improving my coping mechanisms. I feel that if I had carried on going there I would have ended up back in hospital anyway.

Medication

I have tried most medications over the years and it must be highlighted that schizophrenia is a

Annie Moon

biological dysfunction and in the main needs chemical correction in the form of medication. Ultimately, it is not something that you can control by will power, although I have tried! The different medications all had their side effects, ranging from dizziness when standing up to weight gain. I have gained four stones whilst taking Olanzapine; however it's effective in controlling all my symptoms, including the negatives such as lethargy and poor motivation. It also controls my hyperactivity which I get from time to time. I used to get the 'shakes' and twitching on some drugs and my advice would be to keep experimenting with the different medications under the supervision of your psychiatrist until you find one that suits. At the end of the day I have never heard of a medication being free from side effects and you must decide how important it is to be mentally stable in your life, not only for your benefit but for your loved ones that have to put up with you! However, in the early days, I was unable to ascertain whether my negative symptoms were the result of the illness or of the medication's side effects. As my family doctor put it, 'it is all a learning curve', despite sometimes being a long and arduous one, with triumph resulting from good support.

I used to attend a local pool and after a lovely swim I would go in the sauna. It is a standing joke now, between Flick the attendant and I, that she thought that because of my shaking and weight loss, due to being on antipsychotic injections, she would find me dead in the sauna! We had a long

TO SCHIZOPHRENIA AND BACK

chat.

Prejudice and Stereotypes
I find that I can disclose some things to some people. Over the years I have not done too badly with regards the prejudice towards having a mental illness. I must say, however, that the usual length of time for me to get to know somebody and tell them about my schizophrenia is now about eighteen months to two years and that is only when there is a point behind telling them. For example, at university, apart from the faculty leaders and Equality and Diversity department, only a handful of people know and I told them to make a point about stigmatism.
However, after nearly three years on my course and after very stringent vetting by the Occupational Health Department and the General Social Care Council, I came to speak to a senior lecturer who sounded horrified when I spoke about my illness. She wondered why, when she was running the course, she didn't know about me. I explained that my details were on the UCAS form when I applied for the course as well as a statement of needs being sent to her by the Equality and Diversity's Mental Health Advisor- she said 'It would have been nice to be informed'. I cried on and of for days as this was the only form of discrimination that I had come across that kicked me in the pit of my stomach. I had worked so hard to get where I was despite the medication

Annie Moon

and the illness. I thought that I would be ejected from the course. I thought she's not heard of me because I have not given any cause for concern. I met with this person a week later, face to face, and they seemed caring and genuine and put their reaction down to 'surprise'. I feel no animosity towards this person; they helped me with an assignment plan and hopefully changed their view of a 'schizophrenic' on meeting me.

I have been told that I shatter all the stereotypes of someone with schizophrenia. Stephen, a dear friend, said that I had done this for him and he gave me permission to be a 'Social Worker Monday to Friday and a Schizophrenic at the weekend'. He told me how he would tell his friends all about me as he was so shocked about the difference between the public stereotype and me. After a while he settled down and now we say 'who cares!'

At the end of the day, once spoken about, it is old news and the people who are prejudicial are not your friends and you should not waste your precious time worrying about what they think - you could always join me on my awareness crusade!

You should never feel ashamed of who you are. If people don't like you then it only matters if you feel something for those people yourself. I'm not saying put barriers up, what I'm saying is are those people your 'real' friends?

I have recently come across prejudice in the work place, towards a member of the public. Sometimes under stressful conditions people use black humour to alleviate their tension. I would recommend mental health awareness training if this seems to be the case. It would seem to me that you cannot punish these people when they don't know any different and may not have had the same educational opportunities as yourself.

Activities Giving Structure to the day
I found it hard going at the day hospital. My way of reintegrating into society was through the use of college courses, voluntary work and physical activity.

I would at first sign myself up for courses that I had no hope of completing. I was struggling to keep off the sofa let alone do a full time college course. After dropping out a few times, a good friend advised me to try short courses in something that I had an interest in. I followed this advice by doing six weeks, then twelve weeks, etc. After four years of doing this I had qualified in most complementary therapies including massage, aromatherapy, Indian head massage, reflexology and clinical reflexology. I also gained medical secretarial skills, hairdressing skills and so on.

I did feel frustrated at home and so decided after many years of contemplation to study for Social Work. It has filled the void. I now feel fulfilled with ambition and new friends of all ages. I could not have done this if I hadn't rehabilitated myself with the gradual build up of courses and the commitment issues surrounding them. The biggest shock at attending the University was not the work but the fact that everybody had a different accent. I loved and I enjoyed listening to people with different dialects.

My voluntary work has been based around the courses that I have undertaken; I am a voluntary complementary therapist at a local hospice when I'm not engrossed in studies. I have also helped out at the Citizens Advice Bureaux, undertaken administrative work at the hospice and set up and co-run a mums and tots for charity.

The physical activity involved cleaning and ironing for a few friends as well as my walking and swimming.

The whole process enabled me to physically and mentally manage my future. I would, as I have said before, thank God for what I've got and say 'I know that you've got a plan for me' e.g. fate.

I do say to people that everyone has choices in their lives; it's up to them to make the right ones. I would say, however, be thoroughly informed before making those choices. One CPN said to me never make a decision in anger, always wait until you are well or calm before it becomes a regrettable decision. I value this advice as real words of wisdom.

Chat Room

Since becoming computer literate on one of my many courses at college, I have discovered a schizophrenia web site; it offers all sorts of information and advice and the chance to communicate with people in a similar position to

TO SCHIZOPHRENIA AND BACK

you be they parents, children, spouses or sufferers themselves. There is a wealth of knowledge for everyone and it's address is:-
www.schizophrenia.com
Please visit it and you don't have to be that computer literate to follow the different topics.
I've found that over the years I've forgotten passwords etc. but you can always log in again.
I asked the users of this site if they had any questions about the physical/mental and social effects on the sufferer and their close ones. I have dedicated chapter eight to those people.

Questions and unfounded theories of my illness
IS IT
- My abnormal EEG's?
- The extra bits of white matter on my MRI scan?
- Temporal lobe epilepsy?
- Viral as I usually develop cold sores around an episode?
- Because I breast fed for too long?
- Sleep deprivation?
- An old head injury from when I was knocked unconscious in a road traffic accident whilst riding my bike at age 14years?
- Due to being hypnotised during a stage act?

Who knows? There are no definite known causes for schizophrenia; maybe if there were we would be one step closer to curing it. I have spent too much time trying to be given a different diagnosis in the bid to dismiss this 'label' that I myself have stigmatized. I have felt unfit, due to the label, to integrate into normal activities in society. For example, my husband said that he may have to work away for a few days. I was well at the time but I felt it necessary to tell my CPN, despite the fear of my children being taken into care, who wondered what all the fuss was about.

TO SCHIZOPHRENIA AND BACK

CHAPTER SEVEN

REHABILITATION

CARE PLAN 2004

MEDICATION

Currently taking OLANZAPINE 10mg as a maintenance dose.
Annie has agreed with Psychiatrist that she can increase this up to 20mg/day if she begins to experience symptoms of her mental illness.

AREAS OF RISK

Has experienced suicidal ideation and some degree of planning when unwell i.e. has had thoughts of throwing herself under a train or off a motorway bridge. Has made no attempts to act on these, however- when unwell has a history of walking onto the moors in response to psychotic ideation, sometimes with letting death overtake her.

OTHER AREAS OF IMPORTANCE FOR THE CLIENT OR WORKERS

➢ Upset by her elder son's behaviour at present being aggressive and difficult at the moment. Has been arrested for a public order offence and has been suspended from school on several occasions.
➢ Neglected by her mum as a child.
➢ Brothers death (Jan 13th 2001)
➢ Historically she has appeared vulnerable to deterioration in her mental health after the school holidays.

THE EXPERIENCES THAT CAUSE ME STRESS

➢ Difficulties with son
➢ Preoccupation with brothers death when unwell
(not normally a problem when well)

MY STAYING WELL PLAN INCLUDES:

✓ Walking
✓ Listening to music (gives rhythm to thoughts)
✓ Company, having people around me
✓ Time out in the conservatory
✓ Writing
✓ Keeping diaries

TO SCHIZOPHRENIA AND BACK

CHANGES THAT I OR OTHERS AROUND ME NOTICE IN MY HEALTH ARE:-

- Becomes irritable
- Sleeping difficulties
- Becomes weepy when listening to music
- Hears doorbell and knocks at the window when there's nobody there
- Sees shadows
- Sees people (dead brother and mother)
- Withdraws from contact with others, draws curtains, does not answer the door
- Hears voices
- Feels hypersensitive to noise/ touch
- Feels 'floaty'/ 'liquidy'
- Avoids eye contact, appears withdrawn.

Annie Moon

I WOULD LIKE THE FOLLOWING PEOPLE TO BE NOTIFIED SHOULD ANY SIGNS THAT I AM BECOMING UNWELL BE NOTICED:

- ✓ HUSBAND
- ✓ CPN
- ✓ PSYCHIATRIST/GENERAL PRACTITIONER

Action outlined below to be taken:

➢ Husband will ring CPN if he becomes aware that Annie is becoming unwell.
➢ CPN may need to monitor the situation by communication with Husband as Annie tends to avoid contact with services if unwell
➢ Assessment by Consultant Psychiatrist or covering psychiatrist may be necessary if risks cannot be managed at home or in the respite facility

NEEDS/ PROBLEMS

1) Management of risk
2) Management of symptoms when they arise
3) For Annie to be able to live her life as she chooses

TO SCHIZOPHRENIA AND BACK

GOALS

1) Maintenance of Annie's safety
2) For her to be able to maintain stability in her mental health.
3) For her to be able to achieve her goals

Annie Moon

PROBLEM ONE

Problem/ need

At times when Annie experiences deterioration in her mental health- becoming hallucinated, deluded, losing touch with reality- her risk factors may become significant.
During episodes of illness she has had suicidal ideation and has a history of walking off onto the moors to await death.

Goal/ expectation

To maintain Annie's safety during episodes of illness.

Plan

CPN to make ongoing assessment of risk and safety issues in the context of the impact on her safety of any psychotic ideation

CPN to follow up assertively to monitor risk issues in the event of concern being expressed by Annie or her Husband. Withdrawal from contact with services may indicate relapse in mental illness.

Admission to hospital in order to maintain safety may be necessary if Annie is unable to engage in making a plan to minimise any risks if she is unwell.

CPN will liaise with Annie's husband in order to gain feedback on her mental health if she is

TO SCHIZOPHRENIA AND BACK

PROBLEM TWO

Problem/ need

When becoming unwell, Annie often feels that she needs 'time out' from the home situation in order to help her cope with her symptoms.

Goal/ expectation

To assist Annie to cope at these times, in order to avoid full relapse.

Plan

Annie can gain some respite from the situation by spending time on her own in her conservatory.

Annie may spend time at the respite facility if there is a room available if she needs time away from home. Her CPN must assess her mental state prior to her entering this facility, with regards to risk factors i.e. her ability to maintain her own safety. If placed at the respite facility, Annie must inform staff where she is going if she goes out and when she expects to be back. If she goes missing whilst at the respite facility, staff must inform her husband; CPN and police if she is not at home, or the Mental Health Team is unavailable.

Annie Moon

PROBLEM THREE

Problem/ need

At times Annie finds it difficult to cope with the symptoms of her illness and the impact it has on her life.

Goal/ expectation

For Annie to achieve her goals and potential.

Plan

Annie has been referred for Cognitive Behavioural Therapy in order to discuss these issues and to help her explore further coping strategies.

Annie may also discuss these issues with her CPN

CPN to visit regularly in order to monitor her mental health and offer the opportunity to explore any stressors which may impact on her mental health.

Annie may increase her dose of OLANZAPINE up to 20mg if she becomes aware that her mental health is deteriorating.

Annie is to see her Consultant Psychiatrist regularly in her out patient's clinic for review of her mental state and medication regime.

TO SCHIZOPHRENIA AND BACK

CHAPTER EIGHT
CONSULTANT PSYCHOLOGIST

Psychological Intervention

Annie was referred to the Psychological Therapies Team with a request for Cognitive Behaviour Therapy.

Cognitive Behavioural Therapy (CBT) is a psychological therapy that is based on the theory that it is not events or experiences that determine how we feel and behave, but that it is our thoughts about them, or how we interpret the events and experiences. CB therapists work with their clients to enable them to identify unhelpful thoughts or interpretations that lead to feelings of distress and/or behaviours that keep their problems going.

Therapy is led by the client, in that they: decide the problems that they want to work on; identify what they would like to achieve from taking part in therapy; and that the unhelpful thinking styles and behaviours are identified by the client. The therapist asks the questions and suggests structures that help the client to understand the inter relationships between their thoughts (cognitions), behaviours and emotions. The advantage of this approach is that it allows clients to devise and 'own' the strategies to cope with difficulties. These strategies can therefore be used independent from therapy. Such an approach is empowering for the client as it allows them to manage their own recovery.

Assessment

Annie identified the problems that she wanted to work on as:

- Hallucinations – seeing ghosts of dead relatives and hearing knocks at her door and people walking around her house when she knew there was no one there. Annie reported that she found these experiences very distressing and that in the past they had led her to leave her house risking her safety.
- Spiritual beliefs, which had previously led to Annie lying on the moors in poor weather conditions (waiting for god to take her).

Annie reported that her behaviours had caused a great deal of stress for her family and that she felt embarrassed about her past behaviours, particularly because the police had chased her on one occasion. She said that, although she had not experienced the spiritual beliefs for some time, she was afraid that she would experience them in the future and put herself at risk again.

Annie's goals for therapy were:

1. To be able to recognise early signs of

psychosis and develop less risky coping strategies.
2. To reduce disruption to life caused by hallucinations.

We agreed that Annie's name would be placed on our waiting list for therapy. The waiting list was approximately three months at that time and Annie was keen to begin working in therapy as soon as possible. We therefore arrange a further meeting to identify things that she could do whilst waiting for therapy.

In discussion about seeing shadows and hearing noises Annie came to the conclusions that distress caused by these experiences led to her looking for strange occurrences and therefore seeing more distressing things. This heightened her distress and made her want to escape from the home. She also felt more spiritual at these times and this combined with Annie's perceived need to escape led to doing things like going on to the moors which was potentially dangerous.

When examining the events that had happened around the times that she had heard noises and seen shadows, Annie noted that she had tended to have these experiences when several other stressors were affecting her. It was agreed that it was possible that these experiences were reactions to stress rather than to something that could harm her.

Annie agreed that when she heard noises or saw shadows she would practice regarding them as reactions to stress rather than as something threatening. She also identified alternatives to going on to the moors when she became distressed.

Therapy

Annie reported that she had hardly seen any sinister shadows, nor heard noises in the house that had distressed her, in the three months since we'd last met. She also stated that she had found safer ways of coping with stress. Annie had achieved a great deal on her own in the past three months. She had also identified some other problems that she wished to work on:

- Annie said that she was self-conscious around large groups of people and felt as if everyone knew about her mental health difficulties and were judging her negatively because of them. She stated that this was a particular problem on the course that she had recently begun, particularly when discussing mental health issues.
- Annie also reported that when she felt self-conscious she would sometimes experience images of traumatic experiences which she had suffered in the past (such as of being chased by the police, and of being forcibly injected when she was a patient in a mental health ward).

- Continued fear of relapse.

We agreed to another six one hour sessions to work on the new problems Annie had reported.

When discussing Annie's past events, Annie was able to recognise some of the factors that contributed to more recent distressing experiences. Annie requested that therapy did not dwell on childhood trauma and focussed on more recent experiences. However Annie's more recent experiences of using of mental health services were discussed.

Relapse Prevention

Although relapse prevention often gets 'tagged on' to the end of therapy, it appeared that fear of relapse was maintaining Annie's anxiety and making relapse more likely. Annie was able to identify the early warning signs and devise strategies (psychological, behavioural and pharmacological) that she could use if she experienced any of these signs.

Self Conscious Thoughts and Feelings

Annie identified the situations she was in and thoughts that she had when she began to feel self-conscious. With this information she was able to identify the triggers for self-conscious anxiety and

Annie Moon

to be ready to challenge the negative thoughts if they occurred. We also discussed Annie's experiences of people since being involved with mental health services.

It was hypothesised that Annie's feelings of being watched and judged were a consequence of her being observed by family, ward staff and CPN in order to prevent her engaging in anything that might lead to her being harmed. This role of "the person being cared for" did not fit well with Annie's caring for her family and working in a caring profession. This uncomfortable feeling, combined with memories of behaviours that she now felt embarrassed by, increased her self-conscious behaviour. Added to this was the knowledge that many people feel self-conscious in the first tem of a new course.

We agreed to monitor the intrusive images to see if they reduced as the self-consciousness reduced.

We agreed to discontinue therapy after the six sessions. Annie felt that she'd achieved her goals and was confident that she could use the strategies she'd developed to deal with problems, should they arise in the future. I shared her view, as Annie appeared both resourceful and insightful in therapy.

I have spoken to Annie on a couple of occasions over the past two years since therapy.

TO SCHIZOPHRENIA AND BACK

Characteristically she has asked my advice about something, discussed it briefly and then arrived at the answer herself.

DRD

CHAPTER NINE

NEW CAREERS

After undertaking many courses to find some sort of structure for my life, I found that after four years of courses I had no real prospect of financial gain when it came to coming off benefits. I applied to undertake a degree in social work. I had thought of this many years ago whilst I was still nursing but had never actually followed it through.

I couldn't believe it when I received the letter informing me that I had a date for an interview. I was so worried about discrimination and even thought that the rehab team would say derogatory things in the privacy of their office. I thought they would say things like 'who does she think she is?' I don't care so much these days about what people might think of me for the things that I do. I do care, however, that they see me as a good person. This fear is not just a paranoid schizophrenic fear as during my working life I came across professionals saying just that about a woman who had nothing, had hit rock bottom and wanted to turn her life around by training as a dentist. The professionals said just that, 'who does she think she is?' What gives people the right to judge others, surely that lies only with our maker?

I had to tick a box on the application form for university, about my mental illness. I also had to

TO SCHIZOPHRENIA AND BACK

undergo Occupational Health screening. I saw the mental health advisor for the university's equality and diversity department and they gave me a procedure list to assess me for any help or special needs that I may require to help me to complete the course.

Annie Moon

This was the process:-

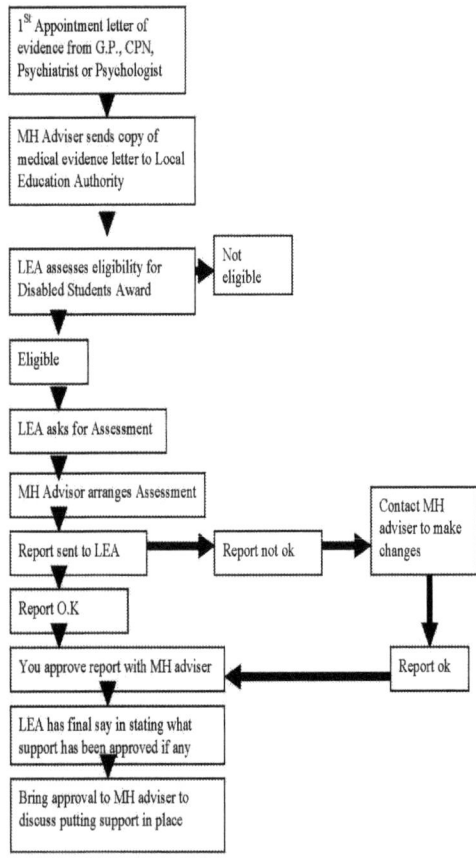

TO SCHIZOPHRENIA AND BACK

After I went through this process the following document was formulated to send to the head of the course to advise them of my learning needs. The contents of the document would make it sound as though I shouldn't be fit to study. I have, however, managed so well with the help of equipment, such as a laptop and photocopying facilities, that my stress has been managed and this has negated the need for submitting PMC (personal mitigating circumstances) forms. I didn't want to be treated any differently and so I have not used the PMC form for any of my assignments, however they are there should I be genuinely ill and need them.

A. STUDENT DISABILITY AND BACKGROUND

General
Annie was diagnosed with schizophrenia in 1995. Her mental health need is classed as severe and enduring.

At times of relapse her symptoms can severely affect her day to day living, and she can experience auditory, visual and olfactory hallucinations and disturbance of thinking. Annie explains that since she has changed her medication, the number and severity of relapses has been significantly reduced. However, relapse can still occur and Annie estimates that this can happen every 3-4 months. Her recovery is now quick and she can return to every day tasks within a week. However after a period of relapse she can experience tiredness, emotional sensitivity and some social withdrawal.

During periods of remission, she experiences the negative symptoms associated with schizophrenia, such as very poor concentration, low motivation, impaired short term memory functioning and lethargy.
Annie manages her mental health well, and is well aware of her 'warning signs' for when a relapse may be imminent. At these times she contacts her CPN and then must go to an environment where she feels comfortable such as her home.

PREVIOUS EDUCATION/EMPLOYMENT
Annie has undertaken several courses (complementary therapy, medical secretary course) and worked on a voluntary basis at a hospice prior to starting at university.

The document then outlines the course delivery and assessment, listing things such as number of hours taught, assignments and their word counts, information about number of days in placement etc.

Facilities and support used to date are recorded; support available to me was also noted i.e. out patients' appointments and involvement of my CPN.

TO SCHIZOPHRENIA AND BACK

My study strategies were highlighted; they included:-
- ✓ Annie will start work early to avoid stress
- ✓ Will plan and organise travel into university as this can cause undue stress
- ✓ If relapse imminent will follow pre-arranged action plan; phone her CPN and go to a familiar place.
- ✓ When reading makes copious notes on every chapter to aid memory
- ✓ Will discuss readings, wherever possible, to cement understanding and memory.
- ✓ Uses a diary for all day to day tasks as well as planning study time.

To enable me to reduce stress in the public area of the library and also to help with the times I may be ill and unable to get to university, it was recommended that I receive help with book costs and photocopying. A laptop and printer, as well as financial help towards internet access at home, were recommended, so that I could have access to the university's intranet. Because I have trouble concentrating at times a Dictaphone was suggested.

Other help, such as extensions to coursework deadlines and extra time in exams, was available should I need it. Extra tutor support for the odd ten minutes was recommended, however this has not as yet been necessary. It was recommended that placement tutors should be aware of my needs on a strictly need to know basis and should be aware that, after a very short relapse or warning signs, I may be tired for a few days afterwards due to medication.

The document included notes for the lecturers providing them with guidance when teaching a student with mental health needs.

The Local Education Authority has provided an excellent service and I will enjoy paying every penny of my council tax when I am working so that another disabled student has the same opportunities that I have been given.

My occupational health clearance didn't come until the second half of my first year. Due to the stress, I disclosed my label of schizophrenia to a placement worker, she told her manager and I was in tears in the office. Nobody could have prepared me for how they were going to speak to me. The first thing the manager said was that she had absolutely no problem with me and if she had I would have been in the office before now. They kept it confidential, I did have to fill in a risk assessment and I was given the task of photocopying the whistle blowing policy- I often wonder if there was some connected reason for this. The staff were all very professional and supportive of each other and I am still in touch with them. I received a glowing report and was

TO SCHIZOPHRENIA AND BACK

really made to feel part of the team.

I have six months left before I finish my course. I may have already said this but I am no longer ashamed of who I am, the sense of achievement I have has given me my self worth back, along with the comments of some professionals.

Self worth should not be underestimated when dealing with rehabilitation.

CHAPTER TEN

CONCLUSION

MY COPING MECHANISMS THAT MIGHT HELP OTHERS

✓ **LISTEN TO YOUR BODY**

When you start pacing, grinding your teeth or twitching, you may be becoming agitated. When you start finding fault with other people, especially your loved ones who can not normally do anything that would annoy you- then you are probably irritable. When you reach for the chocolate or a glass of wine or are tired a lot you are probably stressed. When you need to go to the toilet more often, you may be nervous. I can now relate to these symptoms whereas at one point they would overtake me and my anxiety levels would cause the fight or flight syndrome and I would be off in some psychotic haze on the moors because I hadn't managed my symptoms very well. Now when I recognize these symptoms I telephone my CPN and take extra medication and do some of the activities below.

✓ **CLOSE THE CURTAINS**

TO SCHIZOPHRENIA AND BACK

I do this when I become paranoid and start 'scanning'. When I scan my eyes never stop, I have a heightened sense of awareness, I notice how bright every object is and I notice their symmetry, my brain repeats the scanning of each object, I start to see shadows and outlines of people at the window and I hear knocks and the doorbell ringing when there's nobody there. If I do look in one spot for more than a few seconds my vision 'zings' in my head; by this I mean that whatever I am staring at has a darkened outline, eventually going black and I get a noise in my head- the 'Zing'.

To stop this I close my curtains otherwise I feel that evil spirits are trying to get into my house to harm my family. I have closed the curtains recently and found this extremely therapeutic; although I didn't have any visions I could hear knocking at the window and the doorbell ringing when there was nobody there.

✓ **WRITE**

I found this to be very therapeutic at the start of my illness. My dear friend Ruth told me that if I wouldn't talk to anybody then I should put my feelings down in a book. I was suspicious of everyone except my children. I felt that there was a conspiracy against me and that God wanted me to go to him. By putting it all in my diary, in more lucid moments I would let the professionals read it- it helped a great deal with my diagnosis. Eventually I found that I could talk to the professionals instead. Until this time- and it took me years to develop the trust, the diary was a source of comfort- if anything I felt that if I did die then my family would know about my life and what I was thinking- morbid I know but there you go!

✓ **PAINT**

Having a hobby is a good thing- you don't even have to be good at it! I have goals; I find that having set myself goals gives me something to work towards. I treated myself to all the equipment needed to paint watercolours and acrylics. I even drew and painted a picture of one of my dad's boats. They put it up in their lounge amongst other more fitting ornaments. When I went round to see them I told them that I really appreciated them putting it up and reassured them that I wouldn't be offended if it went in another room a bit more out of site! My aim is to have works of art both by me and my sons on the wall going up the stairway. The ambition is there- this has been a work in progress for about five years' now- but it is something to do for fun. However there have been times when I've been so focused on my art work that when I've stopped I've had some symptoms of the schizophrenia.

✓ **WALK WHEN ANXIOUS TO THINK THINGS THROUGH**

TO SCHIZOPHRENIA AND BACK

I've worn shoes, boots and trainers out walking. When I get the urge, I've just got to walk it off!!! I walk through towns, cities, up country roads and over moors. When I'm ill I take off on my own at any time of the day or night. I don't recommend that. Cognitive Behavioural Therapy has made me change my pattern of just going off. It was very difficult to do at first and I didn't always get it right. I would start sending text messages instead of saying nothing- this caused alarm so I would leave a note but because I was ill and didn't always make sense this too would cause alarm. The last time I felt the urge to go off I asked Stephen my friend if he could put a stressed out mum up for the night. After going round and speaking to him and having a good natter I wanted to go back home. I did this and took extra medicine which worked a treat.

Walking with Todd or friends gives you safe talking and thinking time. There is never the need to fill every moment with conversation, when you're comfortable with somebody silence is fine. Being at one with nature is very calming and sometimes gives you a spiritual feeling when considering the beauty surrounding us.

Plus walking is a good form of exercise to help with the weight gain that accompanies medication. It also releases endorphins, chemicals to make you feel good. It also staves off depression. Not bad for something that's free.

One way I tell friends who have trouble in their life, when they come for a walk with me, is to rate on a scale of 1-10 how they feel. After a very traumatic time Stephen said 1, 1 being the worst; after our walk I asked him again, he said a good 9. Try it, it really works.

✓ **SWIM**

Swimming is good when you are well, for something to do and a good form of exercise. However I've found that when I am becoming unwell then it is too public. I have to communicate with people and this has long since been a 'no no' for me. When you are alright then doing it makes you feel alive! One of my happiest memories was when I was pregnant with my second son. Whilst on maternity leave, I would go swimming for twenty minutes each day during the week. I was so healthy and happy- however my waters did break in the pool, not very nice, I know, for the other swimmers- it was taken care of.

✓ **DIARY MANAGEMENT**

My short term memory is so bad that I can never remember what I had for my previous meal or if I'm not myself I forget that I've got the cooker on and my speciality is burnt pizza!

TO SCHIZOPHRENIA AND BACK

Friends are amazed that I remember their confidences in detail. A friend was amazed that I had not been to his house for a while but I remembered an ornament he had- I commented on where it was- he said that it had been moved months ago and that my long term memory is very good.

I was finding that all my present usable memory (RAM!) was taken up with just functioning. I had to undertake my own portage exercise where I needed to think about the steps needed to be taken just to wash up. I had to think about making a cup of tea in great detail e.g. turn the tap, put water in the kettle, turn it on etc. This left me with no memory space for things such as the children needing special items for school or special assemblies. This was so distressing for me that I began writing everything that I needed to do in a time management diary. I put in things such as wash my hair, vacuum the floor as well as important appointments and activities with the children, even brushing my teeth. I then went on to put in things about asking friends how they went on with their activities- as I would put in when they needed support for hospital appointments etc. This strategy has proved to be invaluable. I tick all my activities when they have been completed and this gives me a sense of achievement- it means that I haven't laid on the settee all day, I have actually done something. Now I don't need to put in activities like brushing my teeth. I put in deadlines that I set myself for assignments, meetings, bills and all activities, especially those with the family. Even though I don't keep a thoughts diary at the moment, I do keep a medicine record; this is just 'O' for Olanzapine and then the dose i.e. 10-20mg depending what I take as I this is a sliding scale depending on my mental health. Other medication is recorded, for example sleeping tablets and Lorazapam, a benzodiazepine which I take on very rare occasions for agitation. Thanks to medication and diary management I have my life back. I have re-learnt how to organise myself- maybe I never had this skill in the beginning and I was approaching life in a very chaotic manner. I have managed to see projects through to the end and was described by a very dear and kind lecturer Shirley, as a 'completer finisher'; apparently this is a management term.

✓ **FRIENDS**

Friends are so important and can be more supportive than some family members. Any new friends are not necessarily told about my illness, as when I'm ill I usually don't answer my phone or the door so they do not see or hear me ranting. After a very long getting to know you period,

TO SCHIZOPHRENIA AND BACK

usually about one to two years, I slip an explanation in that I sometimes don't communicate because I have schizophrenia. Instead of dropping this in at the beginning, it allows people to get to know you without any stigma. Some friends have said 'that explains a lot' when I have told them.

I have friends that I have known for years and they have been there for me when I have needed to talk and vice versa.

I did put a strain on my friendship with Mark a few years ago. I was relying on him too heavily and afterwards realised that he didn't need my stress as well as his own from family and life in general. I texted him and told him that I loved him and thanked him for everything; I suppose it was a goodbye as I was going to meet my maker. Afterwards I found out that he had done a lot of ringing around to involve services because he was worried. He didn't speak to me for twelve months and when I saw him at a carnival, he said that I should take a long hard look at myself. Needless to say I've never bothered him since when I don't feel myself. We still meet up for our annual Christmas drink and a meal, but I don't see much of him now, especially with my course and work placement; however we do text each other now and again.

Annie Moon

I did think that I had a friend in someone right at the very beginning of my illness. She was suffering with depression and I remember talking to her about my worries- she asked me not to talk about it as it was making her worse. I thought about this, she was suffering with severe panic attacks and there was I trying to compare notes of other symptoms! I admired her for her honesty and thought more about how she must be feeling. I can relate this to another friend and nowadays I telephone my CPN or the Evening Advice Line for someone who is trained at listening and I know that they have their professional support network to cope with their stress. I told my Consultant Psychiatrist that I let my CPN do any worrying now and not my friends or family.

✓ **CHAT SITE**

I went on the schizophrenia chat site years ago, just to 'listen in' on the e-mails. When I was psychotic, I began posting (putting my own questions and chat on the site). The people on there were so supportive and helpful; they were in the same situation as I was. When I was well I found that I didn't need to go on. There were some very poorly people from all over the world on that site, yet some very caring and helpful ones too. I remember worrying about starting my social work course and worrying: if I was prejudiced about me, what are other people going to think? One man from the U.S.A more or less told me to 'get a grip', that I wasn't the only schizophrenic in

TO SCHIZOPHRENIA AND BACK

the world and that as long as I'm stable there was no reason why I shouldn't do it- he had and was in a good, well paid job. This really made me take stock as I was becoming insular with my thoughts and was paranoid about what other people thought.

I also asked the people on the website (which has a site for family members as well) about things such as playing the guitar and dieting- that was a big issue with most of the people on the site- the medication had made us a load of fatties! (Although one crass comment made by a professional said that nobody forces you to put the food in your mouth!) I also asked them what they would like me to cover, topic wise, in this book.

The Chat site is an excellent resource for any schizophrenic as long as you don't get hooked and end up on the computer all day and night, neglecting your house and family and giving up good old fashioned fresh air.

✓ **HOW TO COPE WITH PARANOIA**

I find that despite all the coping mechanisms that I have in place, the only thing that will stop my paranoia is medication. I would love to put down some natural remedy, as I have tried allsorts. I did find that spending five hours on the moors in the middle of winter one night did help while it passed as I find it comes in waves. However it does return unless you are taking the correct medication- this is my account, other people may differ. It is a horrible feeling and it can turn me into a very nasty, critical person inside my head- somebody I don't like when well.

✓ LISTENING TO MUSIC

This is excellent. However I try not to play the same music over and over again as in the past, despite giving my thoughts a rhythm to stop paranoid thoughts and ruminating, it can fire you up or make you suicidal. There's nothing I love more than to relax to Celine Dion. However I know of a few people who, if they play it too often, feel suicidal if they are not well anyway (this is not just concerning people with schizophrenia). My advice to someone who says that they feel this way when listening to music is TURN IT OFF or listen to something else. I love a good sixties song which is very up beat, however my brain goes into overload after a while and I may then need to change the tempo to a soul song. There are times however when 'silence is golden'.

✓ AVOIDING THE TELEVISION

At times I have thought that the script writers for the soap operas on television are in my

TO SCHIZOPHRENIA AND BACK

community and are listening to what I say and repeating it in their story lines! Of course, when well, I know this is nonsense.

Daytime T.V has its place but if it's at the expense of your home or family then it is a problem. Try turning it off for a day- you'll be amazed at what you get up to and what you get done.

My Consultant Psychiatrist told me to stop watching too much television- I realised on reflecting over our conversation, that I was actually living a 'television life' i.e. watching Judge Judy, chat shows etc. and letting it creep into conversations and actions. Watching television on your own can be a very isolating experience. Now if I need to get out of the house (of course I realise that not all people can do this especially if they have agoraphobia) then I will go to do some work at the library to have other people around but not necessarily have to engage in conversation. To get out of the house I did try line dancing too!

✓ **LEARNING TO TAKE A JOKE**

I still have problems understanding jokes. I've often seriously wondered if I have some form of autism. I've been described as seeing everything in black and white with no shades of grey. I do take things very literally, but living with my husband has taught me not to read too much into things- a problem I still have. I do absolutely love slap stick comedy with the likes of Jim Carrey and now I like Dustin Hoffman in comedy roles, especially the film 'Meet the Fockars', sooooh funny!

I feel sad that I can't laugh at jokes and some rude ones that friends send me over the Internet I just find distasteful as well as finding ones at other people's expense sometimes just nasty.

If you are in the same boat as me, I would just say not to take things too personally. I have managed this fairly well over the years, maybe not as well as I should have but this may be due to the paranoia of the illness. I can let things ride now and it helps to talk things through, if not with your friends or family then with your CPN or Social worker, Doctor, anybody to put things into perspective.

I came across prejudice against a woman who had mental health problems. She was described by the people concerned as the 'crazy lady'. This was in a work place with professionals who should have known better. This incident really upset me so I talked it through with somebody and they said that some people when under pressure use 'black humour' to alleviate that stress. This explanation really helped as I was horrified when it was going on. I did advise the people concerned that they could do with undertaking mental health awareness training.

TO SCHIZOPHRENIA AND BACK

✓ KNOWING WHEN TO TALK

I consider myself a very private person (when not writing books!) For a long time my Consultant Psychiatrist and others would have to prise conversation out of me. I never ever spoke to my parents about anything and as a result I had a stunted social awareness which hindered me in society when I was younger.

When my Consultant came to my home recently I didn't want to let her in. I did however and spoke to her. She needed to know that I would be safe. Of course you may hold back on what you disclose for fear of having to go into hospital. However if you talk before it becomes out of control your symptoms can be managed. I cannot say this strongly enough- you may feel that people are laughing at you or judging you; now I think so what. What's more important: feeling better by communicating? Or would you rather end up committing suicide or maybe even homicide for those people who might act on their paranoia?

✓ LEARNING TO TRUST

I have taken a long time, over twenty years to learn how to trust. I still don't like speaking out in public because you never know who's listening in. If I do speak in public I try to put the spotlight on

Annie Moon

the other person as I don't like anybody knowing my business unless they specifically ask. I always make sure doors are shut so that nobody can hear a conversation. I also worry about 'chatter' being picked up on the home telephone by the police. I am I suppose amongst many who are concerned over the threat of terrorism and sometimes I think all telephones are tapped, as I knew somebody whose relative worked at a telephone monitoring centre and am aware of their anti terrorism tactics with regards to checking for key words in phone conversations.

To overcome this when I am ill, I just don't use the phone! When I am well, if there is a slight niggling suspicion I just say 'so what!' 'Have they nothing more interesting to do than listen into my chit chat to friends?'

When it comes to professionals it was hard at first because there were so many people coming and going throughout my care in hospital- being a very private person anyway it was such a struggle to disclose my thoughts to the Doctors and Nurses at the hospital. I was sure they were laughing at me and judging me. I had delusions, hallucinations etc. around this. I would tell one person all my business then I would have a new worker. I felt devalued that I had put trust in these people for them to dismiss me onto somebody else. Since having a CPN from the rehabilitation team, despite me having had three which I don't think is too bad, I have taken over ten years to trust them and to

TO SCHIZOPHRENIA AND BACK

feel that I can ring up and speak to anybody be they CPN or Social Worker. It didn't help that for a long time my messages were not getting through and considering I only ring when I really need them I became upset and paranoid, devalued and on my own. I must say that for the last couple of years there must have been a shake up because my messages do get through now. If this book is read by professionals then my helpful tip would be to ensure that your messages are recorded and passed on as this will reduce suffering and maybe even save lives.

My other tip to professionals would be to introduce their client/patient/service user to the team early on so that they feel comfortable speaking to them on the phone or at the door if they are called out. This could be a problem with manpower however if those patients who are just coming into the service realise that you work as a team and not just one patient one worker then it may help with early intervention. I feel that with maturity comes the ability to ask for help. This may sound corny but there are so many leaflets given to you in the early days, maybe one outlining the team and its members might help after all they have boards on hospital wards with nurses pictures and who they are, why not psychiatric services?

✓ **LEARNING HOW TO RELAX**

My methods started out when my birth mum told

Annie Moon

me to take a deep breath in and hold it for ten long seconds, then slowly breath out she said that it was like taking a valium (diazepam)! When I was first admitted to hospital I used this all the time- goodness knows what people thought as they saw my chest puffing out and my face going blue! But it worked.

My next attempt to find ways to relax, involved the sounds of nature from different compact discs with soothing noises on them. This worked too.

I've tried yoga, pilates. I would say find what suits you. I find now that talking to someone helps, by discussing what is making you tense. Also the walking as mentioned. Recently I had to do some motorway driving- I couldn't stay off the loo for two weeks thinking about it! I even went jogging to get rid of some of nervous energy- that worked but the best solution was to face my fear and to 'just do it' as one of my ironing customers recommended. Once I had faced my fear I became relaxed again and ready to face a new challenge. When you're tense it stops you from getting on with life, you mull things round in your head trying to find alternative solutions and sometimes you may catastrophise over fears e.g. I'm going to die on the motorway. The best way to prevent you from simply avoiding your fear, I find is to confront it head on and then you've done it and hey and you may find that it should never have been a big deal in the first place. I even bought a satellite Navigation system to find an alternative route- the motorway was not so bad.

At the end of the day if you have exhausted all your possibilities and you cannot relax and it means preventing a relapse in your condition discussing medication with your doctor for help at these times may be necessary if you haven't already done so.

Never feel ashamed of having to take medication, it took me absolutely years of relapses to finally not be ashamed.

✓ **KNOW WHEN NOT TO TAKE THINGS LITERALLY**

This is one of my problems and I'm sure that I am not alone with this one. When I was a young student nurse as discussed earlier I followed Sisters directions and told a patient she couldn't eat unless she came to the table- I took the Sister's words literally; upsetting everyone in the process. All I can say on this- (because I still do it!) is to ask the person involved what do you mean? My husband said one time that he wished that I'd died on the moors. I took this literally, but what he was saying was that he was stressed out and couldn't cope.

A professional would say why do you I want to work, you're acting like a single person, and

Annie Moon

you've got a family? I took this as holding me back, stopping me from doing what I wanted but I think what they actually meant was they were worried about the effects of working and extra stress on my mental health and ultimately my family. I thought that they thought that I was a danger to the public again a sign that societies stigmas and discrimination have spilled over into how I saw myself.

Always ask the person to elaborate on what they mean, even if it's after a few days of you mulling it around in your head- nip it in the bud because it can hold you back from recovery or remission however you see it.

My husband once said to me about a football match- 'they're letting them in', I said 'oh that's nice of them', thinking that they were letting the crowd in for free- he actually meant that his team were letting the other side play by not defending them- maybe my gripe should be with the English language!!!

TO SCHIZOPHRENIA AND BACK

CHAPTER ELEVEN
Mental Health Social Exclusion and Employment

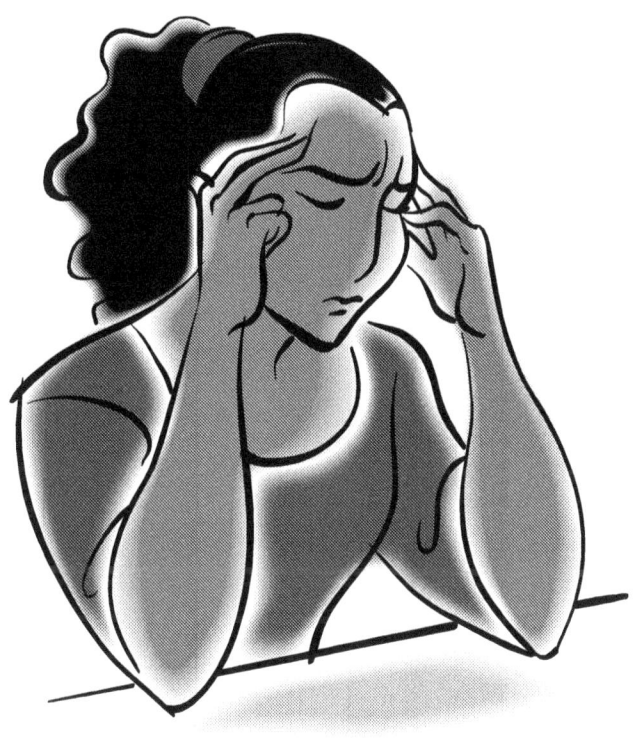

Before reading this my main uncertainty for returning to work was of a financial nature- what if I gave up my benefits, started a new job and was then ill again. In the U.K the New Labour Government has devised benefits to cover this at

Annie Moon

present. If you do start work you must inform the benefits agency at jobcentreplus who will suspend you benefits at the same level for up to twelve months. If you have to give up work during this time, you may resume the same level of benefits. The following is an assignment that I submitted for my BA (Hons) Social Work course in 2007. It is itself in three chapters.

TO SCHIZOPHRENIA AND BACK

ABSTRACT

The area covered within this assignment is that of mental health, social exclusion and employment. It discusses the prejudices, stigmas and discrimination for those people/ service users that have a mental illness and are seeking to return to employment.

Current research has been drawn from also included are the social workers codes of conduct and NOSSW key roles with regard to the social workers input.

The report document Mental Health and Social Exclusion (ODPM 2004) has been examined. From this and other relevant material I have discussed how society including social workers and other partnership agencies can work together to promote social inclusion for those people with a mental illness wishing to return to work.

Myths that people with mental illness don't want to work are dispelled and the research discussed highlights that the matter is quite the opposite and not only do newly diagnosed service users want to work as with early intervention to minimise the social decline of the patient/ service user, but also those who have been ill for up to twenty five years

Discrimination and stigma are discussed and I have included relevant current research and studies that highlight what the problems are for the mentally ill returning to work and also how these barriers can be worked through to gain employment and educate the public especially employers about mental illness.

Government and professional documentation has been used including the Disability Discrimination Act (DDA 2005) has been included including the National Service Framework, NICE guidelines NOSSW and GSCC codes of conduct including key roles in order to discuss how the social worker may help their service user by empowering, and advocating for them. Also research has been shown that despite clients wanting to work professionals often don't provide the information available maybe because they don't know and maybe it's because their client may be clinically stable and they put them off working to maintain their mental health.

During the summer whilst undertaking my research project, I was fortunate enough to attend an education teaching session for employers about mental health and employment run by Headstart (now Rights to Work) this literature has been included in my assignment and to be aware of it is a valuable resource for any social worker to not only help their clients but also to reduce stigma and discrimination by educating the public.

TO SCHIZOPHRENIA AND BACK

CHAPTER ONE

Within this assignment I will discuss the literature available relating to mental health, social exclusion and employment.

In this chapter I will be addressing current research and literature around the subject including stigma and discrimination encountered by those suffering with mental illness wishing to return to work.

Social exclusion is the term used to describe what happens when people or areas are excluded from essential services or every day aspects of life that most of us take for granted. (Communities and Local Government 2006)

In spring 2003, the Prime Minister and the Deputy Prime Minister asked the Social Exclusion Unit (SEU) to consider what more can be done to reduce social exclusion among adults of working age with mental health problems. One of the questions was that of employment.

The report Mental Health and Social Exclusion (ODPM 2004), found that only 21% of people with long-term mental illness were employed- the lowest of any disabled group. More than a million who wanted to work were jobless and the cost to the economy of missed employment opportunities was £23bn a year. But less than four in ten employers said they would employ someone with a mental health problem compared to six in ten for someone with a physical disability (Batty 2004) from (Taylor Nelson Sofres (2003).

The National Institute for Mental Health in England (NIMHE) spearheaded a five year plan in the same year to tackle the stigma surrounding people with mental health problems.

The SEU identified five possible reasons for those suffering social exclusion these include:-
- Stigma and discrimination. Many people fear disclosing their condition even to family and friends let alone employers (Manning and White 1995 in SEU Report).
- Low expectations
- Lack of clear responsibility
- Lack of ongoing support to enable them to work
- Barriers to engaging in the community (ODPM 2004)

The report goes on to explain the barriers to employment such as:-
- Lack of motivation and self esteem resulting from their illness
- Fear that work will lead to deterioration in mental health, when in fact it is likely to help.
- People unaware of the possible support available to them to ease the transition back into work.

TO SCHIZOPHRENIA AND BACK

- Benefits and the feeling of a real threat to their financial security- 37% of the respondents to the SEU consultation identified this as a barrier to returning to work.

Most people who suffer from periods of mental ill health would like to work and yet less than 20% are in employment. For those with a diagnosis of schizophrenia, the unemployment rate is probably nearer to 95% (Grove et al 2005). Grove et al describe losing a job as a

'reckless waste of a life' for sufferers. Kruger (2000) argues that a full recovery may be possible for some people with schizophrenia.

Despite the literature on the benefits of early intervention with regards to recovery rates and employment (Bond et al 2001), research such as the Vermont Study (Harding et al 1987) and a European study (Harrison et al 2001) have produced findings reporting that recovery can be made despite years of illness.

Dr Alan Whitehead (1994) highlighted benefits of work which also reduces isolation and exclusion whilst encouraging a sense of citizenship. These benefits are as follows:-

✓ Regularity

Annie Moon

- ✓ Social and personal contact
- ✓ Daily structure
- ✓ External validation
- ✓ Personal esteem
- ✓ Normality

- ✓ The end of the 'sick note'
- ✓ The chance to move on to possible paid employment.

Despite benefits to work such as reduced anxiety and depression (Department for Work and Pensions 2003), reduced risk of suicide (Lewis and Sloggett 1998) and reduced risk of clinical deterioration for those with schizophrenia (Wing and Brown 1970) and the fact that those who are employed have fewer hospital admissions and symptoms than their counterparts (Brown et al 1958), there is still stigma and discrimination and the fear that if you have a mental illness then you must be an 'mad axe man' (Whitehead 1994).

Not only do those suffering with severe mental health problems encounter stigma and discrimination based on their 'label', they also encounter other forms of social exclusion when it comes to employment such as race, gender, religion and age all compounding the problem despite their being government legislation in the form of Acts of parliament including the Disability Discrimination Act (1995 updated in 2005) and the Race Relations Act (1976).

TO SCHIZOPHRENIA AND BACK

Again more findings on discrimination and stigma with regards to low expectations on the part of mental health professionals also pose a problem (Read 1997; Harris et al, 1997; Webster, 1998). Not only does this compound the problem but it has a negative effect on the self esteem of those service users who may already discriminate against themselves (Duckworth 2001; Carrigan and Watson, 2002)

When barriers are put up by potential or actual employers which is a major issue (Read and Baker 1996) Gates (2000) and Mental Health Foundation (2002), those people who have a mental illness may fail to disclose their condition thereby excluding the help available to them as outlined in the Disability Discrimination Act (1995 and 2005) for the employer to make all reasonable adjustments such as flexible work patterns and any specialist equipment within their remit. Granger (2000) highlighted this as yet another barrier.

There have been articles on 'coming out' about ones disability. Swain and French (2000) under the title 'proud angry and strong' discuss what they call the 'affirmative model of disability. They

address the divide between the disabled and the non-disabled and how their disability has an affect on their lives and social identity, rather than dismissing, denying or re-interpreting ones experiences the affirmation model is 'borne of disabled peoples experiences as valid individuals, as determining their own lifestyles, culture and identity'. It builds on the social model, through which disabled people envisage full participative citizenship and equal rights. Disabled people want a life without structural, environmental and attitudinal barriers and they wish to embrace equality and diversity (Swain and French 2000).

Corrigan (2003) An American psychiatrist said that we should try and change societies views by coming out about mental illness. He does however go on to say that we should not be naïve about this and there will be stigma and discrimination especially in the workplace. He says that family, professionals and advocates should be aiming to change society's attitude. He goes on to say that we should obtain interpersonal, legal and other substantial support for those who step up to the challenge. Corrigan describes this 'coming out' as an 'anti stigma' program.

According to the SEU report on mental health (2004) they highlighted some startling figures; they noted that despite little proportional increase in those adults with psychosis entering back into the workforce their physically disabled counterparts had a significant increase back into employment.

Also in the report during consultation, interviews

TO SCHIZOPHRENIA AND BACK

were carried out and it was noted that those with probable psychosis had fewer formal qualifications, were less economically active, tended not to own their own home, fewer were married or cohabiting and had poorer physical health than those who were not seen as mentally ill.

CHAPTER TWO

Within this chapter I will be discussing ways of promoting social inclusion by examining relevant literature.

Two white papers *'The new NHS'* and *'Modernising Social Services'* were the landmarks for the future of health and social services. They set out a range of measures to drive up quality and reduce unacceptable variations, with services responsible to individual needs, regardless of age, gender, race, culture, religion, disability, or sexual orientation. A First Class Service explained how NHS standards would be:

➤ Set by the National Institute for Clinical Excellence and National Service Frameworks.
➤ Delivered by clinical governance, underpinned by self- regulation and lifelong learning.
➤ Monitored by the Commission for Health Improvement, the new National Performance Assessment Framework, and the National Survey of Patients. (Department of Health (DH)1999)

The National Service Framework focuses on the mental health needs of working age adults up to 65. The DH describe mental ill health as being so common that at any one time around one in six people of working age have a mental health problem, most often being anxiety or depression. One person in two hundred and fifty will have a psychotic illness such as schizophrenia or bipolar

TO SCHIZOPHRENIA AND BACK

affective disorder (manic depression), (DH 1999).

The National Service Framework for Mental Health explain that some people with severe and enduring mental illness will continue to require care from specialist services working in partnership with the independent sector and agencies which provide housing, training and employment. Working partnerships with agencies providing amongst other things employment will be required to address the needs of some people with enduring mental health needs. (DH 1999)

The National Service Framework was developed by an External Reference Group chaired by Professor Graham Thornicroft, from the Institute of Psychiatry, King's College London. The

External Reference Group brought together health and social care professionals, service users and carers, health and social service managers, partner agencies, and other advocates. The National Framework is founded on their work which included research, current issues personal views and knowledge (DH 1999).

The External Reference Group developed ten guiding values and principles to help shape decisions on service delivery. People with mental health problems can expect that services will:

Annie Moon

1.   Involve service users in the planning and delivery of care both on a one to one level or this may be in the form of sub groups which would meet regularly and discuss topical issues and aim to resolve conflict or solve problems.   Their expenses would be reimbursed.
2.   Deliver high quality treatment and care which is known to be effective and acceptable.
3.   Be well suited to those who use them and non-discriminatory.

4.   Be accessible, so that help can be obtained when and where it is needed.
5.   Promote their safety and that of their carers, staff and the wider public.
6.   Offer choices which promote independence.
7.   Be well co-ordinated between all staff and agencies.
8.   Deliver continuity of care for as long as it is needed.
9.   Empower and support their staff.
   10.   be properly accountable to the public, service users and carers.

The National service Framework (1999) Standard One is about mental health promotion. Its aim being to promote health and social services, promote mental health and reduce the discrimination and social exclusion associated with mental health problems.

TO SCHIZOPHRENIA AND BACK

Health and social services should:
- ✓ Promote health for all, working with individuals and communities

- ✓ Combat discrimination against individuals and groups with mental health problems and promote their social inclusion.

Mental health problems can result from the range of adverse factors associated with social exclusion and can also be a cause of social exclusion e.g.

- ❖ Unemployed people are twice as likely to have depression as people at work (DH 1999)

In the document 'National Service Frameworks' The following was discussed:-

Surveys by the Department of Health, MIND and the Health Education Authority (HEA) all report that people feel strongly about mental illness. (DH 1997; Repper et al 1997; HEA 1997). Most people are generally caring and sympathetic, but they are also concerned about the danger which they associate with a very small number of people with severe mental illness. The HEA report *Making*

Headlines (1997) shows that negative media coverage of mental health is widespread. Public education is an effective way of reducing stigma (Wolff et al 1996). The Department of Health through its *Impact* strategy, works in partnership with service users, the Royal College of Psychiatrists, Mental Health Media and the voluntary sector, to provide better information and build understanding among the public. The document goes on to say how the Government has spent over £2.5 million nationally on providing public information and health promotion over 1997/1998 and 1998/99. It says that subsequent standards in the National Framework assess the needs of the mentally ill, however it goes on to recognise that help will be needed in tackling discrimination. It says how Legislation requires organisations to make reasonable adjustments to accommodate the needs of disabled employees (DDA 1996 and 2005). The DDA places a duty on employers to prevent all disabled employees including those with a mental health disability from being placed at a disadvantage.

In 1996 Peter Bates published a ground-breaking study that challenged the assumption that people with mental illness do not want to work. In the study he found that out of 77 day centre attendees questioned, 61% said that they would like to work, despite them having been contact with mental health services for an average of 21 years.

Rinaldi and Hill (2000) studied 127 people who

TO SCHIZOPHRENIA AND BACK

were not working, almost half of them had a mental health problem, 63 (51%), wanted to return to work, including 23 people who reported having been advised not to work by health professionals. In total, 55 people had been given that advice.

In the General Social Care Council's Codes of Conduct (GSCC) (2002 currently in use), in section one, as a social care worker you must protect the rights and promote the interests of service users and carers. This includes:-

1.1 Treating the person as an individual;

1.2 Respecting and where appropriate, promoting the individuals views and wishes of both service users and carers;
1.3 Supporting service users' rights to control their lives and make informed choices about the services they receive;
1.4 Respecting and maintaining the dignity and privacy of service users;
1.5 Promoting equal opportunities for service users and carers; and
1.6 Respecting diversity and the different cultures and values.

The following information is available in Grove, Secker and Seebohm (2005). Seebohm and Secker (1999) carried out a study in Sheffield to find out what service users wanted in relation to employment, training and education. One hundred and fifty six service users took part. The survey questions were answered by ticking a box; however there was provision for any comments. When asked if they were interested in work of any kind only 10% had no interest in any kind of work at all. Participants who were interested in work, education or training were asked the opportunities that they would like to be given. 95.7% wanted paid employment (full time, part time or self

employed). When asked if they had received any kind of help an astonishing 53% said that they had not received any help. Those who had received help were asked to name the source of that help. 30% was from a Community psychiatric nurse (CPN) and a poor 16.7% was from Social Workers. Considering the research on benefits of employment and the codes of conduct for social workers there is an obvious lack of intervention here.

The study highlights barriers to employment as in Table 1.on page 18

The needs highlighted in this research were:-

- Impartial trustworthy advice about benefits from people who understand both the benefits system and mental health and employment issues
- Expert careers advice, again from people with an understanding of mental health and employment issues

- Information about opportunities provided in day centres through talks and written material

- The provision of information in community languages

- **Table 1. Barriers to employment**

Barrier	% (n)
Employer attitudes	83 (129)
Mental health problems	80 (124)
Benefits system	69 (107)
Lack of work experience	54 (84)
Lack of support	53 (83)
Lack of skills or qualifications	51 (79)
Age	50 (78)
Lack of vacancies	49 (77)
Public transport (availability or difficulty using it)	30 (47)
Caring for others	17 (27)
Other	15 (23)

(p.14 Secker and Seebohm, edsGrove 2005)

At the moment mental health services are predominantly available during the day and during the week ideal for the unemployed, however this is not so good for those who need the support once they have returned to work. Although some areas of the United Kingdom have advice lines as part of their community teams and also weekend workers, however maybe more evening workers would benefit the service user who needs extra support whilst working.

The Disability Alliance has published a guide 'The Way to Work' (2005) specifically to help mental health professionals improve the advice they give to service users thinking of returning to work.

The GSCC (2002) codes of conduct part 3 it states that as a social care worker, you must promote the independence of service users while protecting them as far as possible from danger or harm, in relation to employment and mental health this would encompass the following codes:-

3.1 Promoting the independence of service users and assisting them to understand and exercise their rights;
3.2 Using established processes and procedures to challenge and report dangerous, abusive discriminatory or exploitative behaviour or practice.

Also Social Workers must be accountable for the quality of their work and take responsibility for maintaining and improving their knowledge and skills (GSCC Code 6 2002). This is not the case when reflecting back on the research stating that only 16.7% of service users had help from a social worker when asked about employment and training opportunities (Seebohm and Secker 2005). The Social Worker must know their area of

TO SCHIZOPHRENIA AND BACK

expertise and should be aware of initiatives such as 'Early Intervention' and the benefits to service users with regards to employment.

Early intervention services provide community based treatment and support to young people with psychosis and their families, with an emphasis on maintaining normal social roles (DH 2001).

The SEU report (2004) concluded that early intervention is needed to keep people in work.

Figure 2 shows the 'vicious cycle of despondency (p.22), it highlights the problems such as if professionals who are supposed to be the experts in their field, are telling them not to get jobs how hard is it going to be in mainstream society?

Figure 2. The Vicious Cycle of Despondency (Secker, Seebohm and Grove 2005)
Expert professionals say that people with mental health problems are unlikely to be able to work

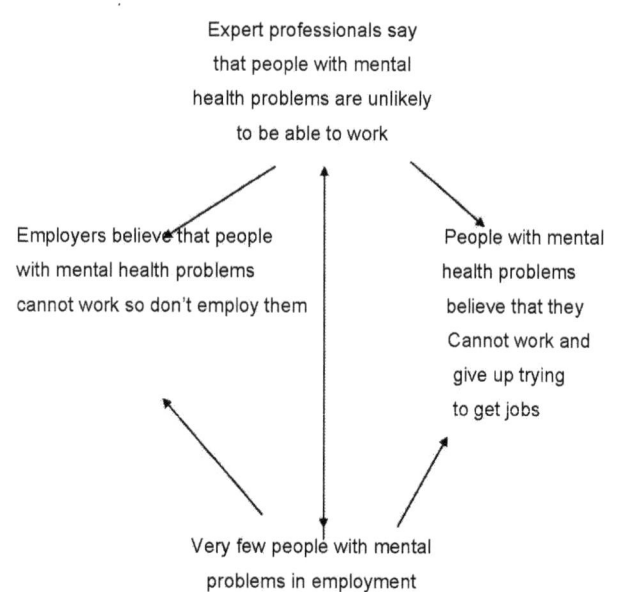

TO SCHIZOPHRENIA AND BACK

CHAPTER THREE

This chapter will discuss literature relevant to mental health and employment. It will discuss topics such as empowerment and anti discriminatory practice aimed at the knowledge available for the role of a social worker, in essence, to promote social inclusion.

'Empowerment is a transformational activity', Adams (2003)

Empowerment may be defined as 'theory concerned with how people may gain collective control over their lives, so as to achieve their interests as a group, and a method by which social workers seek to enhance the power of people who lack it'. (Thomas and Pierson, 1995 p. 134)

Empowerment is rationalistic, that it has links with humanist and existential theory and practice, in that it emphasises self-knowledge and self-control, accepting that people can control their own lives by rational, cognitive means (Adams 2003). However when a service user wants to work, yet as mentioned in highlighted research, not

Only are the professionals demeaning the urge to work but also employers, therefore making it an uphill struggle for both the enlightened social worker and his/her service user. The service user may be empowered by different events or knowledge for example one may feel empowered by something understood and yet another person by getting that job. (Adams 2003).

Self help was re-ignited in the United Kingdom in the 1980's after Solomon's writing in1976. The Wolfendon Report came out in 1978 which emphasised the significance of the voluntary sector in developing partnerships between individuals, informal networks of support, voluntary bodies and the statutory agencies. Much of this is encompassed now in the form of agencies both statutory and voluntary to help those with a mental health disability return to work.

The benefits agency, as part of Labour's New Deal, offer specialist advice at job centres through a disability advisor. They discuss benefits and assist with C.V.s and interview techniques as well as

actively looking for work on the service users behalf. (Jobcentreplus 2006)

Some educational establishments have mental health advisors in the Equality and Diversity department providing disability assessments to claim practical help for those with either mental or physical disabilities (Access Summit 2004).

The Benefits agency, jobcentre and educational

TO SCHIZOPHRENIA AND BACK

facilities promote 'Bridging the Gap' an empowering initiative which allows students to remain on their benefits whilst they study, thereby reducing stress and possible relapse in this context in relation to a mental illness. This is an excellent attempt by the Government to break down barriers and allow the disadvantaged to help themselves. Jobcentreplus (2006)

At a recently attended discussion 'Routes to Work' (2006) (formerly Headstart) spoke about their aim to provide training and consultation to employers to decrease the stigma and increase mental well being

In the workplace. In July 2006 Headstart (a service that supported people with mental health issues) and Jobmatch (a service that supported people with other disabilities) merged into 'Routes to Work'.

Referrals do usually come via social workers or CPNs however there are drop in centres locally which are advertised in public buildings such as libraries, day centres and out patient departments. There is however a waiting list locally of a couple of months. Once referred the service user will get a key worker who will undertake an assessment followed by a plan of action.

Routes to Work have their own reasons of what

often stops people with mental illnesses getting jobs these are:-

❖ Fear of losing benefits
❖ Fear of not managing a new course/ voluntary work/ job- Wanting to try something out before committing to it.
❖ Unsure of skills if they haven't worked for a while

❖ Not knowing what's available
❖ Needing to build confidence
❖ Needing a bit more support to make a change
❖ Unsure of how and if to disclose their illness to an employer- fear of stigma. (Routes to Work 2006)

The agencies mentioned all act as advocates for the service user they also refer them on to other agencies such as welfare rights or the Citizens Advice Bureau. This is a requirement of the National Occupational Standards for Social Work (NOSSW key role 3 unit 10.3 2006)

As mentioned earlier not only do they work in partnership with other agencies such as community psychiatric rehabilitation services but they also support the service user by visiting potential employers with them and negotiating their need to an employer. They find information for them and help to build up their confidence ready for when they have interview or start a job

TO SCHIZOPHRENIA AND BACK

or a course. They negotiate with the clients (service users) and 'bounce' ideas off them.

The document goes on to talk about the 'Best Practice Model' with which the Employer Consultant delivers. During the consultation process Routes to Work aims at reducing stress in the workplace and by this promoting mental health. Their training package includes mental health awareness, stress awareness, time management and the Disability Discrimination Act. They discuss recruitment and retention strategies, support in the workplace assistance to build their own policy for managing mental health in their workplace. They give useful contacts and ongoing advice.

The training on mental health awareness run by Routes to Work for employers gives them the opportunity to find out about diagnosis's, signs and symptoms, practical advice and about stressors in the workplace and how to reduce them.

CONCLUSION

Within this assignment I have discussed the social exclusion around in our society focused on the problems of stigma and discrimination

that arises when somebody with a mental health problem specifically those with a severe illness tries to gain employment.

The benefits of work have been outlined for those service users. Myths have been dispelled that these people don't want to work, actually they do and evidence shows that this is a major aspiration for many people with a mental illness.

Government legislation has been discussed with reference to NICE, National Frameworks, DDA, NIMHE, GSCC codes of conduct and the NOSSW's.

The final chapter discusses how as a social worker you can aim to empower an individual by being up to date in your field and also about how different agencies namely Routes to Work can re-balance the stigma surrounded by mental health with regards to educating employers.

TO SCHIZOPHRENIA AND BACK

FINALLY

Georgina Sinclair, a member of a poetry group for disabled young people wrote the following poem:-

Coming Out

And with the passing of time
you realise that you need to find
people with whom you can share.
There's no need to despair.
Your life can be your own
and there's no reason to condone
what passes for their care.
So, I'm coming out.
I've had enough
of passing and playing their game.
I'll hold my head up high.
I'm done with sighs
and shame.
(Tyneside Disability Arts 1999, p.35.)

REFERENCES

Access Summit (2004) Joint Universities Disability Resource Centre. *Working together to promote provision for people with disabilities*
St Peter's House, Precinct Centre, Oxford Road, Manchester.
Email: info@access-SUMMIT.ac.uk

Adams R (2003) Social Work and Empowerment 3rd edition. BASW. Palgrave Macmillan: Hampshire

Bates P (1996) Stuff as dreams are made on. *Health Service Journal.* 4th April: 33.

Batty, D and agencies (2004) Guardian Unlimited at:-
http://society.guardian.co.uk/mentalhealth/story/0,8150,1238682,00.html (29/11/06)

Bond, G. Resnick, S.Drake, R et al. (2001) Does competitive employment improve non vocational outcomes for people with severe mental illness? *Journal of Consulting and Clinical Psychology.* 69 (3): 489-501

Brown, G., Carstairs,G. and Topping G (1958) Post-hospital adjustment of chronic mental health patients. *Lancet.* 2: 685-9

Carrigan PW and Watson AC (2002) The paradox of self stigma and mental illness. *Clinical Psychology Science and Practice* 9 (1) 35-53

Corrigan P (2003) Taking Issue. Beat the Stigma: Come Out of the Closet Psychiatric Services at:- http://ps.psychiatryonline.org October 2003 Vol. 54 No.10

Department for Work and Pensions (2003) *Pathways to Work: helping people into employment.* The Stationary Office, Norwich.

Department of Health, (1998) *A First Class Service: quality in the new NHS.*

Department of Health
Website: - www.doh.gov.uk

Department of Health (2001) The *Mental Health Policy Implementation Guide.* Department of Health, London

Department of Health (1997). *Mental health surveys* (DH, London).

Disability Alliance (2005) The *Way to Work-a guide to benefits and tax credits for mental health professionals,* Disability Alliance, London.

Disability Discrimination Act (2005)

http://www.skill.org.uk/info/infosheets/dda.doc

Duckworth S (2001). The disabled person's perspective. *Report on New Beginnings-A Symposium on Disability.* Surrey: Unum Limited

Gates LB (2000) Workplace accommodation as a social process. *Journal of Occupational Rehabilitation* 10 (1) 85-98

General Social Care Council (2002)
Codes of Conduct
www.gscc.org.uk

Granger B (2000) The role of psychiatric rehabilitation practitioners in assisting people in understanding how to best assert their ADA rights and arrange job accommodation. Psychiatric Rehabilitation Journal 23 (3) 215-223

Grove, B., Secker, J. and Seebohm, P (2005) New Thinking about Mental Health and Employment p. xv

Grove, B., Secker, J. and Seebohm (March 2006) What Have We Learnt About Mental Health and Employment? *The Mental Health Review Volume 11 Issue 1*

Harding, C, Brooks, G. Ashikaga T et al (1987) The Vermont longitudinal study of persons with severe mental illness: Methodology, study sample and overall status 32 years later. *American Journal of Psychiatry* 144(6): 718-26

Harrison, G. Hopper, K. Craig, T. et al (2001) Recovery from psychotic illness: a 15- and 25 year international follow up study. *British Journal of Psychiatry.* 178: 506-17

Harris, M, Bebout RR, Freeman DW *et al*, (1997) Work stories: psychological responses in work of dually diagnosed adults. *Psychiatric Quarterly* 68 (2) 131-153

HEA. (1997) *Making headlines: Mental health and the national press* (Health Education Authority, London).

Jobcentreplus (Including jobcentres and security offices from 30th October 2006) at:-
www.jobcentreplus.gov.uk

Lewis, G. and Sloggett, A (1988) Suicide, deprivation and unemployment: record linkage study. *British Medical Journal.* 317: 1283-1286

Manning, C and White, P.D.,'Attitudes', Psychiatric Bulletin, 19 (1995):541-543

Mental Health Foundation (2002) Out at Work: *A Survey of the Experiences of People with Mental Health Problems Within the Workplace.* London: Mental Health Foundation

Annie Moon

Modernising Social Services: promoting independence, improving protection, raising standards.
The Stationery Office, 1998, CM 4169

National Service Frameworks. Modern Standards and Service Models (Sept 1999) Department of health: - www.doh.gov.uk

National Institute for Clinical Excellence:-
NICE.org.uk

ODPM (June 2004) Mental Health and Social Exclusion. Social Exclusion Report either from:-
http://www.communities.gov.uk/index.asp?id=1127160 (23/11/06) and follow links
or ISBN: 1851127178 Crown Copyright ODPM publications
Race Relations Act 1976
http://www.direct.gov.uk

Read J and Baker S (1996) *Not Just Sticks and Stones: A Survey of the Stigma, Taboos and Discrimination Experienced by People with Mental Health Problems.* London: Mind

Read, J. (1997) What is a good day project? *A Life in the Day* 1 7-11

Repper, J., Sayce, L., Strong, S., Willmot, J. & Haines, M. *Tall stories from the backyard* (MIND, London, 1997).

TO SCHIZOPHRENIA AND BACK

Rinaldi M and Hill R (2000) *Insufficient Concern*. Merton Mind, London.

'Routes to Work' (2006) Powerpoint presentation presented by Kate Reed. Training Consultant.

Seebohm P and Secker J (2005) What *do service users want?* Research details in New Thinking about Mental Health and Employment pp11-18.

Sinclair, Georgina (1999) Tyneside Disability Arts, p.35.

Social Exclusion- Communities and Local Government:-
http://www.communities.gov.uk/index.asp?id=1127160 (23/11/06)

Swain J and French S (2000) Towards an Affirmation Model of Disability. *Disability and Society*, Vol. 15, No. 4 pp569-582

Taylor Nelson Sofres, *Attitudes to Mental Illness 2003 Report* (London, Department of Health/Office for National Statistics 2003)

Thomas, M. and Pierson, J. (1995) Dictionary of Social Work, London, Collins Educational

Webster, A (1998) An unchartered journey. *A Life in the Day* (2) 9-12

Whitehead, Dr A, (1994) The Transition from Work to Employment in Mental Health At Work Eds Michael Floyd, Margery Povall and Graham Watson. Jessica Kingsley Publ:London

Wing, J. and Brown,G. (1970) *Institutionalism and Schizophrenia: a comparative study of three mental hospitals.* Cambridge University Press, London.

Wolfenden, Lord (1978) The Future of Voluntary Organisations: Report of the Wolfenden Committee, London. Croom Helm.

Wolff, G., Pathare, S., Craig, T. & Leff, J. (1996). Public education for community care: a new approach. *British Journal of Psychiatry* **168**, 441-447